INTERNATIONAL BOOK OF DYSLEXIA

INTERNATIONAL BOOK OF DYSLEXIA
A GUIDE TO PRACTICE AND RESOURCES

Edited by **Ian Smythe**, **John Everatt** and **Robin Salter**

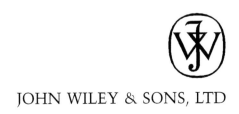

JOHN WILEY & SONS, LTD

Other Wiley Editorial Offices

John Wiley & Sons Inc., 111 River Street, Hoboken, NJ 07030, USA

Jossey-Bass, 989 Market Street, San Francisco, CA 94103-1741, USA

Wiley-VCH Verlag GmbH, Boschstr. 12, D-69469 Weinheim, Germany

John Wiley & Sons Australia Ltd, 33 Park Road, Milton, Queensland 4064, Australia

John Wiley & Sons (Asia) Pte Ltd, 2 Clementi Loop #02-01, Jin Xing Distripark, Singapore 129809

John Wiley & Sons Canada Ltd, 22 Worcester Road, Etobicoke, Ontario, Canada M9W 1L1

Wiley also publishes its books in a variety of electronic formats. Some content that appears in print may not
be available in electronic books.

British Library Cataloguing in Publication Data

A catalogue record for this book is available from the British Library

ISBN 0-471-49646-4

Typeset in 10/12pt Times by SNP Best-set Typesetter Ltd., Hong Kong
Printed and bound in Great Britain by Antony Rowe Ltd., Eastbourne
This book is printed on acid-free paper responsibly manufactured from sustainable forestry
in which at least two trees are planted for each one used for paper production.

CONTENTS

INTRODUCTION
Dyslexia – different contexts, same problems

Ian Smythe and Robin Salter

Whereas Part 1 of this book considered aspects of dyslexia that are related to individual languages, Part 2 focuses on aspects that relate to individual countries. These chapters include discussions of many issues, including those relevant to the education system, public and professional awareness, legislation and policies, definition and terminology and prevalence within the country discussed. Practical issues of identification and assessment, intervention and resources, provisions for children and adults, as well as teacher training, advocacy groups and details of where to obtain help (voluntary and professional organizations) are also given in many chapters. In addition, some authors include further discussions of the language-related issues, such as the language context of the country and aspects of dyslexia difficulties specific to the language(s) used. Although the information provided cannot be totally comprehensive, it can be used as a guide to what is happening around the world, as well as to views and perspectives held by many individuals in a wide range of countries.

When reading all the diverse approaches to dyslexia represented in this volume (research perspectives, teaching methods, definitions, services), it is easy to get lost in the wealth of information and provision available. But, as Steve Chinn, principal of a UK specialist dyslexia school, often says, where is the dyslexic individual in all this?

We should celebrate diversity, of approaches and viewpoints, of policies and practice, but only if it leads to answering the central question: how best can we help this dyslexic person? The formation of this question in terms of 'this dyslexic individual' is deliberate to emphasize the idea that there is no 'one size fits all'. Every dyslexic individual is different. So too is every country, culture and educational context. From these pages there

International Book of Dyslexia: A Guide to Practice and Resources. Edited by Ian Smythe, John Everatt and Robin Salter. ISBN 0-471-49646-4. © 2004 John Wiley & Sons, Ltd.

can be little doubt that dyslexia is an international concern. However, perceptions, aware-ness and understanding within the community, the resources available, whether financial, manpower or teaching resources, will dictate the importance at the personal, school or leg-islative level. Given the perceived importance of dyslexia assessment and support, and the importance recognized at least among some educationalists from different countries and language backgrounds, there is a need for systematic research which identifies similari-ties and differences between these contexts which will aid in the development of appro-priate diagnostic and remediation tools.

LEGISLATIVE SUPPORT

Legislation does not equal provision. As just one example, visitors to the UK are frequently surprised to learn that despite apparent legislative provision, case after case comes before the special educational needs review tribunal of children who are five or even more years behind in terms of their literacy skills and still have not been appropriately assessed or provided with appropriate support.

The framework for provision has been with us for some time. For example, in 1948 the UN General Assembly, in Resolution 217, Article 26, declared that 'Everyone has the right to education. Education shall be free, at least in the elementary and fundamental stages. Elementary education shall be compulsory.' Sadly, that goal has never been met, with large numbers of parents being forced to pay for basic education, both in terms of attendance and for the resources available in classrooms, such as books. Furthermore, in the context of dyslexia, what the Resolution failed to emphasize was the need to make that education appropriate.

By the end of the Jontiem conference (1990), some progress had been made. The Jontiem declarations stated that the individual should 'be able to benefit from educational opportunities designed to meet their basic learning needs' (Article 1), and that 'Steps need to be taken to provide equal access to education to every category of disabled persons as an integral part of the education system' (Article 5). Also included was the statement that 'The focus of basic education must, therefore, be on actual learning acquisition and outcome, rather than exclusively upon enrolment' (Article 4), and this 'should be met through a variety of delivery systems' (Article 5).

By the time of the Salamanca Statement (UNESCO, 1994), which concentrated more specifically on special educational needs, these ideals had expanded to the following:

- every child has unique characteristics, interests, abilities and learning needs;
- education systems should be designed and educational programmes implemented to take into account the wide diversity of these characteristics and needs.

The Salamanca guidelines included a need to take full account of individual differences (Statement 21), adapting to the needs of the child (Statement 28), providing additional assistance and support to children requiring it (Statement 29), identifying difficulties and assisting pupils to overcome them (Statement 31), and offering appropriate teacher train-ing (Statement 42).

However, as shown throughout this book, despite the large number of participants and signatories, and direct and indirect reference to Salamanca in national legislations, imple-mentation in practice is, at best, patchy. Inclusion has meant that, with few exceptions, the dyslexic individual has been taught in the mainstream. Although this is a desirable outcome in a world where 'inclusion' is the buzz word, the role of the specialist centre (such as a private specialist dyslexia school, or a state centre of excellence) should not be ignored. Frequently, these become the source of teaching methods and resources which then migrate to the state system.

It is interesting the way different countries interpret their needs, not only within the Salamanca framework, but also within their own linguistic and cultural context. The diversity of definitions of dyslexia has been discussed elsewhere (see Smythe and Everatt, Chapter 1 in Part 1). The diversity of contributors to this Part, from government officials, to non-governmental organization spokespeople, reveals the range of viewpoints and approaches that exist around the world. All, in principle, follow a similar framework for policy, resources and training (see the chapter on Wales for more details), but interpretation is derived within the context of their own language, funding, culture, political agenda and, of course, with respect to the viewpoint of their education advisors.

Part 2 of the book provides a snapshot of the interpretations found around the world. Obviously, all views cannot be expressed. While England may talk of its Code of Practice which should be a safety net for all dyslexic individuals, the truth is that many still fall through that net, due to diversity of policy interpretation, resource availability, teacher training and funding. Similarly, it is difficult to generalize about provision in the United States, where every state has its own legislation, and one short chapter cannot cover the diversity of provision (or lack of) in that country. What is exciting is to see the way some countries have changed since the first version of this book in 1997. Not only do we see new countries represented, indicating their increased awareness and understanding in the intervening period, but also we see changes in individual countries, such as Hong Kong, where identification has increased exponentially, and resource development and training have been relentless over the past few years.

SAME PROBLEMS, SIMILAR SOLUTIONS

Smythe and Everatt (see Part 1) suggest that the manifestation of dyslexia will depend not only upon the cognitive profile of the individual, but also on the language they use. Dyslexia must be evaluated with respect to an individual's own linguistic, cultural and legislative context. However, at the same time, despite many definitions of dyslexia referring to the single word decoding, most practitioners agree that dyslexia is far more than this. Areas such as study skills, writing at length, organization skills and memory strategies are considered to be important by educators of dyslexics, and are commonly referenced around the world. Fortunately, the desire for practitioners in one country to share their resources with those of another has been demonstrated many times, leading to a spread of ideas and tools. Obviously care must be taken when transferring one idea to another context, but the principle of helping a child write at length may work as well for the dyslexic Chinese child as for the dyslexic Hungarian child.

WHAT'S IN A WORD?

The term 'dyslexia' (or to be more precise 'dislexie') was first used by Kausman in 1883, who adopted the common practice of using Greek or Latin morphemes to develop a new word. The combination of the 'dys-' meaning difficulties, and 'lexis' meaning word, provides a simple basis for common understanding, which many have used and interpreted for their own needs. The term has become a word of universal understanding of the difficulty in the acquisition of literacy skills, and can be found in many languages, translated in many ways. More recently there has been a trend to acknowledge that defining the cut-off criteria, necessary to decide who does, or does not, receive support, is difficult with dyslexia. Disagreements over cut-off criteria and the need to acknowledge an increasing number of specific learning difficulties (e.g. dyspraxia, dysgraphia, ADHD, dysorthographia, dysautographia, to name but a few), many of which can coexist in any one individual, have led to a trend for assessments being made with respect to identifying specific cognitive strengths and weaknesses, rather than making categorical judgements. Dyslexia, therefore, is sometimes referred to as one of many specific learning difficulties (SpLDs). Other countries will use terms such as 'learning disabilities' (the United States and Canada), legasthenie (used by German speakers), while the equivalent term in Chinese (in Hong Kong) is translated as 'reading and writing difficulties'. However, in common use, the term 'dyslexia' and its 'linguistic relatives' (i.e. various forms of translation) remains dominant, and is understood throughout the world by parents, practitioners, researchers and dyslexics themselves.

In this age of the Internet, it can be thought easy to access information. However, it is important to remember that such access is not available to all. Sharing of information can take many forms. Marion Welchman, to whom the first version of this book was dedicated, was an international facilitator. It is hoped that this book will continue that work and provide a valuable resource in terms of information and inspiration to those looking to help the dyslexic individual. Ultimately, such information will hopefully lead to many more dyslexics being given the opportunity to fulfil their potential.

Each author who was asked to contribute to this volume was provided with the same brief. However, each has interpreted it in their own way, with respect to their own understanding, their own views, and their own cultural, linguistic and national context. In comparing and contrasting these approaches to dyslexia, and the responses to the same brief, we may celebrate differences, in the same way we celebrate differences in individuals which can make the dyslexic individual so special.

EUROPEAN DYSLEXIA ASSOCIATION

Reference has been made by a number of countries contributing to this book of the *European Dyslexia Association* (EDA). The EDA was created as a charity under Belgian Statute in 1987 by representatives of eight European countries and has since grown to having 41 member organisations in 28 countries, three of whom are outside Europe.

The aims of the EDA are to assist and develop support for dyslexic people in their educational, social and cultural integration into society; to promote co-operation between parents, teachers and other professionals; to publish news of its activities and to encourage research into causes, diagnosis, intervention and prevention; to carry out comparative studies and to co-operate world-wide with other organizations with similar aims.

A number of conferences have been organized by the EDA in different countries, the latest being the All-European Conference in Budapest, Hungary in October 2003. *EDA NEWS* is published three times a year. Financial support comes three from its members, sponsorship and the sale of its publications.

DYSLEXIA IN ARGENTINA

Maria Jose Quintana

INTRODUCTION

Argentina, a country of over 36 million people with Spanish as the first language, has adopted the international practice of inclusive education, with special needs children being integrated into mainstream schools. However, policies are more concerned with physical or severe mental handicaps than specific learning difficulties. The integration policy in Argentina is outlined in the *Acuerdo Marco para la Educación Especial* (Special Education Agreement Ministerio de Cultura y Educación, 1999). This Agreement states that, 'Special Educational Needs are those experienced by individuals that need extra help or resources not readily available in their educational context to aid them in the process of constructing meaning from the learning experiences set out in the curriculum.' This document sets the baseline for the future and progressive transformation of the Special Educational Needs system in our country. The aim is to develop the quality of public schools in order to make them more inclusive for children with special educational needs. Now, practice has to follow policy.

Within Argentinian legislation and policy there is no official definition or recognition of dyslexia as a distinct area of need. The *Acuerdo Marco* includes the need of dyslexic students within the spectrum of children with special education needs (*NEE: Necesidades Educativas Especiales*), and consequently there is no specific educational provision for students with dyslexia.

The term 'dyslexia' is used by some professionals in the field of education (educational psychologists, psychopedagogists, neurolinguists and speech therapists), but there is a preference for the terms 'Specific Learning Difficulty' (SpLD) and Learning Disability (LD). In a more general way, it may be referred to as 'difficulties in the acquisition of reading and writing' or 'reading and writing problems'.

International Book of Dyslexia: A Guide to Practice and Resources. Edited by Ian Smythe, John Everatt and Robin Salter. ISBN 0-471-49646-4. © 2004 John Wiley & Sons, Ltd.

PUBLIC AND PROFESSIONAL AWARENESS

There is a low level of awareness of dyslexia among the general population and few people understand the extent of the difficulties facing the dyslexic individual. However, increased media attention has helped raise the profile of the subject. Furthermore, in 2000, one whole day (out of a total of four) was dedicated to 'Dyslexia' at the International Neuropaediatrics Conference held in Buenos Aires City. However, one of the key objectives of the newly formed (2001) Asociación de Padres de Hijos con Dificultades de Aprendizaje (APDHA) is to raise public awareness.

Currently, dyslexia is given little coverage in study programmes in universities and teacher training colleges. In general, there is a low level of awareness in the educational community of the difficulties experienced by children with dyslexia.

IDENTIFICATION AND ASSESSMENT

Many schools have a special needs coordinator (SENCO) responsible for liaising between teachers, parents and professionals. Any child noted as having difficulties would be brought to the attention of the SENCO, who would gather appropriate information and liaise with the parents. Together the SENCO and parents would devise the strategies to follow which may include a school-based assessment to define the need for a referral. When no SENCO is available, all the responsibility falls on the classroom teachers, who are not trained in ways to help these children.

If it is considered appropriate, children are referred to free assistance centres within the educational system, to child psychology departments at public hospitals, private professionals or language centres for assessment and/or remediation. A diagnosis of 'dyslexia' depends on the theoretical framework used by the individuals conducting the assessment, but the majority of them will consider it an 'LD'. Usually the school will be informed of the results of their assessment and in the best of cases will be provided with some guidelines for the classroom teacher. A further problem is the small number of reading and spelling tests available in Spanish and that practically none of the specific assessment procedures or tests are validated or standardized in Argentina.

Assessment methods and techniques

A professional assessment conducted by speech therapists, psychopedagogists or neurolinguists considers two aspects:

- reading, writing and spelling;
- the underlying cognitive processes.

Reading and writing assessment includes silent and oral reading, visual and phonological tasks, miscue analysis, metalinguistic abilities and reading comprehension as well as free writing. Spelling is assessed in copy, dictation and creative writing. Observation of written school work results is also important.

Cognitive functions assessment usually includes measures of intelligence, auditory and visual gnosias, global and fine motor skills, graphomotor coordination, attention, memory, laterality, cerebral dominance, linguistic and sequential skills.

The following tests created in Spain or Latin America are used in Argentina:

- Prueba de Comprensión Lectora de Complejidad Lingüística Progresiva (CLP) (Allende);
- Test de análisis de lecto-escritura (TALE) (Toro y Cervera);
- Test exploratorio de Dislexia Específica (Condemarín);
- Batería Woodcock de Proficiencia en el idioma (Español) (Woodcock);
- PROLEC- Batería de evaluación de los procesos lectores en Educación Primaria (Cuetos, Rodríguez and Ruano).

REMEDIATION

There is no specific remediation for learning disabilities in schools. It takes place individually and off the school premises. It may be prescribed by doctors, but it is more likely to be suggested to parents by the special education needs coordinator if the school staff includes one, or directly by the classroom teacher. It is free of charge at public hospitals. It may be completely or partially covered by the social security system or is paid for by parents privately. Parents assume a decisive and central role as they are responsible for the treatment of their dyslexic child.

Remediation methods

The remediation of reading and writing disabilities in the context of an individual treatment will consider: general and specific characteristics of the reading and writing difficulty, the child's strengths and weaknesses, individual learning styles, the emotional aspects and curriculum adaptation as suggested in the *Acuerdo Marco*. The treatment is arranged by the professional conducting the remediation and the school as there are no specific guidelines provided in the referred official document.

Although most schools provide only the minimum of support, and rarely have anyone with specialist knowledge, there are some dyslexia-friendly schools which provide more extensive support for these students. This may include a flexible grading and marking policy, the use of a personal computer, oral rather than written examinations and on very limited occasions the provision of one-to-one tuition. The nature of the support provided depends greatly on the knowledge the teachers or other members of the staff may have on the subject. Educational policy does not set any guidelines on the kind of support children with SpLD should be given.

ADVOCACY GROUPS

I'm the mother of a 12-year-old boy. I've known he was dyslexic since he was nine years old. He seemed to be a very smart boy until he got to school. Something was wrong; he had difficulties with reading and writing, even maths. During the first three years in school, teachers said he was immature and that he needed more time. When he reached third grade my husband read an article in English, and recognized our son's condition. We then had him tested and diagnosed as 'dyslexic'. He started special instruction with an educational therapist. After two years he could read and write better, but this did not reflect in his school marks. The school he attended never got really involved in knowing what dyslexia is.

When looking for a new school for him, it was evident that no school knew much about dyslexia; they are not aware of how to detect it or even how to manage these children in school. I felt that my child was suffering more from a teaching disability than his own dyslexia.

During that time I met many parents who had the same problems. So in 2001 we started an association.

Asociación de Padres de Hijos con Dificultades de Aprendizaje (APHDA)

APHDA is a parents' group and its aims are:

* to promote awareness and understanding of specific learning difficulties so that proper identification and intervention can be made promptly;
* to help schools to train teachers in the detection and management of learning difficulties;
* to support parents through various means, including arranging meetings with professionals related to education, to lectures to parents and teachers on reading and writing difficulties.

REFERENCE

Ministerio de Cultura y Educación (1999) *Acuerdo Marco para la Educación Especial* (Documentos para la Concertación, Serie A, N° 19), Buenos Aires.

ORGANIZATION

APHDA (Asociación de Padres de Hijos con Dificultades de Aprendizaje)
García Mansilla 2860
(1644) Victoria
Buenos Aires
Argentina
Tel./Fax: 5411 4745-8788
Email: aphda@hotmail.com

CHAPTER AUTHOR

Maria Jose Quintana
Acassuso 673
1636 – La Lucila
Prov. Buenos Aires
Argentina
Email: mjosequintana@hotmail.com

DYSLEXIA IN AUSTRALIA

Paul Whiting

THE PRINCIPAL ORGANIZATIONS

The Australian contribution to the first version of this work (Salter and Smythe, 1997) was written by Yvonne Stewart, who founded the specific learning difficulties movement in Australia. Owing to her work, autonomous SPELD organizations were set up in all states of Australia, and in New Zealand and Fiji. A national organization, AUSPELD, was also established. For many years, these have been the main organizations representing the interests of people with dyslexia.

These organizations are supported in a variety of ways: state governments supply some funds in recognition of the service provided to the community and the education systems, usually to support a telephone advisory service for parents and others. Other funds come from the sale of books, Christmas cards, and the efforts of volunteers, but most rely on membership fees. Across Australia, there are more than 5,000 members of SPELD organizations.

SPELD NSW was established in 1968, and another organization, the Association for Children with Learning Difficulties (ACLD), was established in 1972. This organization continues, though with broader concerns than dyslexia, as Learning Links Inc. In addition, there is the Victorian-based Learning Difficulties Australia (formerly Australian Resource Educators' Association), a professional association for educators in the field of learning disabilities, difficulties and differences. It has a council of members from five states of Australia comprising university lecturers, consultants and tutors. They publish the only ongoing journal for dyslexia in the country, the quarterly *Australian Journal of Learning Disabilities*.

Geographically Australia is a large and diverse country, with a population of 19 million spread over an area approaching 3,000,000 square miles. This has made it difficult for state-based or national organizations to meet all the needs of parents, so regional parent support groups were formed, initially at the suggestion of SPELD and with its support in New South Wales. In 1988, however, another organization was formed in that state to

International Book of Dyslexia: A Guide to Practice and Resources. Edited by Ian Smythe, John Everatt and Robin Salter. ISBN 0-471-49646-4. © 2004 John Wiley & Sons, Ltd.

assist these support groups. This is the Learning Difficulties Coalition. There are currently 19 parent support groups in the state of NSW.

SPELD and similar organizations offer services mostly aimed at the parents of children with dyslexia, though some offer services to adults. Services typically include a telephone help line, referrals (to tutors, educational psychologists, speech pathologists and other relevant professionals), assessments, a specialist library, sales of books on dyslexia-related subjects, a newsletter for members, conferences, and some training courses. In 2002, for example, SPELD in the state of South Australia offered 21 training courses for parents and professionals. Some organizations (for example, SPELD Victoria) also offer some tutoring services.

Referrals are made after a consultation, most frequently to formal assessment through an educational psychologist, then to tutoring and supportive literature. Referrals are also sometimes made directly to speech pathologists, occupational therapists, and optometrists. Some organizations also offer counselling services.

ASSISTANCE FOR DYSLEXIA

Most parents and others concerned with dyslexia must seek assistance outside the school system. This is because school systems either do not recognize dyslexia as a specific learning difficulty or have inadequate resources to help every child. This is understandable, when it is considered that the proportion of children potentially requiring additional assistance will approximate 7 per cent (estimates have ranged from 2 per cent to 11 per cent, and even higher) (Andrews *et al.*, 1979; Louden *et al.*, 2000). The result is that many families cannot afford the assistance available through organizations like SPELD. From a national planning perspective, it would be preferable to provide adequate teaching services in schools, as the Australian Business Council (for example) estimated a few years ago that poor or non-existent literacy costs Australia $3 billion per year.

GOVERNMENT PROVISION

In most states of Australia, government Departments of Education do not directly recognize learning disability, dyslexia or specific learning difficulties except by inference. They therefore do not offer targeted help. However, government school systems are increasingly emphasizing effective early teaching of literacy and numeracy skills (Elkins, 2001). This is part of an attempt to reduce the need for expensive support services later in a child's education progress. In addition, most states attempt to intervene early through Reading Recovery programmes (Clay, 1993a, 1993b) for children who do not begin reading successfully by the end of the first year of school. This programme is effective for the majority of students who are slow to begin reading, but is not effective for dyslexic students (called by the NSW Department of Education and Training (DET), students with 'significant learning difficulties') (Center *et al.*, 1995). Some SPELD organizations note that the greatest difficulty their clients have is that dyslexia is not recognized as a lifelong disability that requires ongoing support and is not able to be remediated by short courses.

In two states, NSW and Queensland, school systems offer the help of a support teacher for learning difficulties. Currently there are nearly 1,200 of these teachers in NSW. These teachers, sometimes allocated to one school but often shared between schools, must assist with the identification and assessment of learning difficulties of all kinds, must plan, implement, monitor and evaluate programmes for students with learning difficulties, and provide either in-class support or short-term intensive withdrawal programmes, as well as providing training and development for classroom teachers (see, e.g. NSW DET, 2001). These services are rarely adequate for the needs of dyslexic students. Only NSW has a district and state-level infrastructure to support these teachers. In addition, NSW has 35 support classes for reading, each taking six students for one term with a further term of in-school follow-up.

In South Australia, a centrally-based Learning Difficulties Support Team provides professional development, information and advice to groups of parents, Learning Assistance Programme volunteers, School Services Officers, individuals and groups of teachers. The service covers pre-school to Year 12. Professional development is also negotiated to suit individual sites. Topics include information about characteristics of learning difficulties/learning disabilities, inclusive methodology, effective teaching practices and ways of supporting and accommodating students in the different learning areas.

Where there is not direct support (e.g. from a Support Teacher), states rely wholly on the regular class teacher to modify the curriculum appropriately for dyslexic students. Needless to say, in many cases the modifications are not made, because teachers just do not have the knowledge and time to make them. In some cases, advice is available from learning difficulties consultants in the State Office of Education.

Parents or adult dyslexics thus find that they must seek help outside the education system, and may obtain it from Irlen Dyslexia Centres, Samonas Sound Therapy, Educational Kinesiology, Paediatric Physiotherapy or Occupational Therapy, Behavioural Optometry, Feuerstein Instrumental Enrichment (Kozulin *et al.*, 2001), Biofeedback, etc. Many of these approaches offer to correct underlying processing deficits leading to dyslexia. More conventional approaches that are widely used are *Alpha to Omega* (Hornsby and Shear, 1993), *The Writing Road to Reading* (Spalding and Spalding, 1969); *Visualising and Verbalising* (Bell, 1986), *Auditory Discrimination in Depth* (Lindamood and Lindamood, 1975), or one of the many phonics-based approaches such as THRASS (Ritchie and Davies, 1996), or *Discovering Reading through Sounds* (Lamond and Whiting, 1992), etc.

TECHNOLOGY AND DYSLEXIA

The Internet has, to a great extent, internationalized dyslexia so that few approaches are unique to Australia. Many of the approaches listed above have come from other countries. The same is true of technologies that have not until now been widely used in Australia. SPELD has made available to groups and individuals a computer-based program from the UK, the *Touch Type, Read and Spell* program, which has materially assisted many dyslexics (Whiting and Chapman, 2000). An increasing number of such programs are available, claiming to assist dyslexics. Other tools, such as the Reading Pen (a hand-held scanner that reads words and phrases to the student) (Whiting, 1999), text readers such as the Kurzweil 3000, *Read and Write* (www.texthelp.com), hand-held spellers such as the *Franklin Spellmaster,* portable keyboards such as *Alphasmart* (www.alphasmart.com), brainstorming and organizational programmes such as *Inspiration,* and dictation and text-prediction programmes are all just beginning to be used. *Textease,* a talking word-processor, is used by some 'good teachers' in Victoria for primary students mainly, as is the spelling programme *WordShark*. Unfortunately, their utility is not widely recognized, even by educational authorities.

SPECIAL PROVISIONS (REASONABLE ACCOMMODATIONS)

Many school systems in Australia offer special provisions to students who are shown to be dyslexic and whose performance without the specified provision is impaired. These provisions include extra time in examinations, use of a reader and/or writer for examinations, use of a laptop computer, examination papers printed on individually specified coloured paper, separate room for examination or larger print for exam papers.

HELP FOR ADULT DYSLEXICS

There is little specific assistance available for adult dyslexics in Australia. The only formal provision comes through the Further Education (TAFE) system, and many of the 109 campuses in NSW offer some provision for learning disabilities instruction, though it is usually offered under some other category of service (such as 'neurological disabilities'). Many campuses offer classroom instruction in literacy, but this is not acceptable to most adults whose prior experiences in classrooms have been so disappointing. In any case, such instruction is not intended for dyslexics. Other states of Australia offer services to people with disabilities, but it is not clear that this specifically includes students with dyslexia. Assistance in the form of special provisions is available to dyslexic students in universities (Mungovan *et al.*, 1999).

Adults seek help from sources that happen to be publicized in the media, and may find such help in private centres such as those referred to above.

RESEARCH

Research into aspects of dyslexia is being conducted in a number of Australian universities, and some operate centres that include learning disabilities (dyslexia): at the University of Queensland, the Sir Fred and Eleanor Schonell Centre; at the University of Sydney, the Evelyn McCloughan Children's Centre; at Macquarie University, the Special Education Centre; and at Newcastle University, the Special Education Centre. In addition, in each state there is one or more Irlen Dyslexia Centre, concerned mainly with assessment and treatment of visual perceptual difficulties resulting in dyslexic symptoms.

From the above lists, it will be seen that there is not much research directed specifically at dyslexia. One reason may be the difficulty of recruiting dyslexics for research when school systems do not identify dyslexia. However, there is some research of good quality, and mention should be made of the internationally recognized research on language processing in reading disabilities emanating from the University of New England in NSW (e.g. Byrne *et al.*, 2000), from Macquarie University (e.g. Coltheart *et al.*, 1996), and that on visual perceptual difficulties from Newcastle University and the University of Sydney (e.g. Robinson and Foreman, 1999; Robinson *et al.*, 2001; Whiting and Robinson, 2001), and the University of Wollongong (e.g. Conlon *et al.*, 1999).

LEGISLATIVE PROVISIONS

Australia has no protective legislation such as that of the United Kingdom and the United States. However, in 1992 the Australian government passed the Disability Discrimination Act which offers protection against discrimination for people with all kinds of disabilities, including those that result in them 'learning differently'. An example of this category of disability would be 'a person with autism, dyslexia, attention deficit disorder or an intellectual disability' (Tait, 1995). The Australian Human Rights and Equal Opportunity Commission states that learning disability is covered by the Disability Discrimination Act (www.hreoc.gov.au/disabilityrights).

The application of this legislation was tested in 2000 before the Human Rights and Equal Opportunity Commission. In that case the Commission found that, 'The complainant, . . . suffers from dyslexia. Expert evidence . . . satisfied me that the complainant's dyslexia amounted to a "disability" within the meaning of the Disability Discrimination Act 1992.' The party complained against, which had denied the complainant special provisions in examination, was fined. This has been a recent and important landmark in the struggle to have the needs of dyslexics addressed in Australia. A case has yet to succeed where the complaint is that a student has been denied appropriate educational provisions. This author's understanding is that school authorities have settled all such complaints out of court, thus evading the possibility of adverse findings.

Without specific legislation, however, Australia is in a more difficult position than either the UK or the USA, where a requirement for specific educational provision is supported by legislation, and does not have to be argued on the grounds of discrimination.

REFERENCES

Andrews, R.J., Elkins, J., Berry, P.B. and Burge, J. (1979) *A Survey of Special Education in Australia: Provisions, Needs and Priorities in the Education of Children with Handicaps and Learning Difficulties.* St Lucia, Qld: Fred and Eleanor Schonell Research Centre, The University of Queensland.

Bell, N. (1986) *Visualising and Verbalising for Language Comprehension.* Pasa Robles, CA: Academy of Reading.

Byrne, B., Fielding-Barnsley, R. and Ashley, L. (2000) Effects of preschool phoneme identity training after six years: Outcome level distinguished from rate of response. *Journal of Educational Psychology*, 92, 659–667.

Center, Y., Wheldall, K., Freeman, L. and McNaught, M. (1995) An evaluation of Reading Recovery. *Reading Research Quarterly* 30, 240–263.

Clay, M. (1993a) *Reading Recovery.* London: Heinemann.

Clay, M. (1993b) *The Observation Survey.* London: Heinemann.

Coltheart, M., Langdon, R. and Haller, M. (1996) Computational cognitive neuropsychology and acquired dyslexia. In B. Dodd, R. Campbell and L. Worrall (eds), *Evaluating Theories of Language: Evidence from Disordered Communication.* San Diego: Singular Publications.

Conlon, E.G., Lovegrove, W.J., Chekaluk, E. and Pattison, P.E. (1999) Measuring visual discomfort. *Visual Cognition*, 6(6), 637–663.

Elkins, J. (2001) Learning disabilities in Australia. In D.P. Hallahan and B.K. Keogh (eds), *Research and Global Perspectives in Learning Disabilities.* Mahwah, NJ: Lawrence Erlbaum Associates.

Hornsby, B. and Shear, F. (1993) *Alpha to Omega.* 4th edition. London: Heinemann.

Kozulin, A., Feuerstein, R. and Feuerstein, R.S. (eds) (2001) *Mediated Learning Experience in Teaching and Counseling.* Jerusalem: The International Center for the Enhancement of Learning Potential.

Lamond, J. and Whiting, P.R. (1992) *Discovering Reading through Sounds.* Sydney: Evelyn McCloughan Children's Centre.

Lindamood, C.H. and Lindamood, P.C. (1975) *Auditory Discrimination in Depth.* Allen, TX: DLM Teaching Resources.

Louden, W., Chan, L.K.S., Elkins, J., Greaves, D., House, H., Milton, M., Nicholls, S., Rivalland, J., Rohl, M. and van Kraayenoord, C. (2000) *Mapping the Territory: Primary Students with Learning Difficulties: Literacy and Numeracy.* Vols 1, 2 and 3. Canberra, ACT: Department of Education, Training and Youth Affairs.

Mungovan, A., Allan, T., England, H. and Hollitt, J. (1999) *Opening All Options.* Universities Disabilities Cooperative Project (NSW). Also at http://student.admin.utas.edu.au/services/alda/options/index.html

NSW DET (2001) *Who's Going to Teach my Child?* Sydney: Department of Education and Training.

Ritchie, D. and Davies, A. (1996) *THRASS Special Needs Pack.* London: HarperCollins.

Robinson, G.L. and Foreman, P.J. (1999) Scotopic sensitivity/Irlen syndrome and the use of coloured filters: A long-term placebo-controlled and masked study of reading achievement and perception of ability. *Perceptual and Motor Skills,* 89, 83–113.

Robinson, G.L., McGregor, N.R., Roberts, T.K., Dunstan, R.H. and Butt, H. (2001) A biochemical analysis of people with chronic fatigue who have Irlen syndrome: Speculation concerning immune system dysfunction. *Perceptual and Motor Skills,* 93, 486–504.

Salter, R. and Smythe, I. (1997) *The International Book of Dyslexia.* London: World Dyslexia Foundation.

Spalding, R.T. and Spalding, T. (1969) *The Writing Road to Reading.* New York: William Morrow.

Tait, S. (1995) *The Users Guide to the Disability Discrimination Act.* Geelong: Villamata Publishing Service.

Teaching Handwriting, Reading and Spelling Skills. http://www.thrass.com accessed 6 March 2002.

Whiting, P. (1999) Report on the trial of the reading pen. *Australian Journal of Learning Disabilities,* 4, 36.

Whiting, P.R. and Chapman, E. (2000) Evaluation of a computer-based program to teach reading and spelling to students with learning difficulties. *Australian Journal of Learning Disabilities,* 5(4), 11–17.

Whiting, P.R. and Robinson, G.W.L. (2001) The interpretation of emotion from facial expressions for children with a visual subtype of dyslexia. *Australian Journal of Learning Disabilities,* 6(4), 6–14.

ORGANIZATIONS

SPELD Victoria Inc
494 Brunswick St
North Fitzroy
Victoria 3068
Australia
Phone: (61 3) 9489 4344
Email: speldvic@bigpond.com.au
Website: www.vicnet.net.au/~speld

SPELD South Australia
298 Portrush Rd
Kensington
SA 5068
Tel.: 8431 1655
Email: info@speld-sa.org.au
Website: www.speld-sa.org.au/index.html

SPELD NSW Inc
7 Acron Rd
St Ives
NSW 2075
Tel.: (02) 9144 7977
Email: speldnsw@bigpond.com
Website: www.speldnsw.org.au

SPELD (Tas) Inc
250 Murray Street
Hobart
Tasmania 7000
PO Box 154
North Hobart 7002
Tel.: (03) 6231 5911
Email: speldtasmania@bigpond.com

Dyslexia-SPELD Foundation WA (Inc)
PO Box 409
South Perth WA 6951
Tel.: (08) 9474 3494
Email: speld@opera.iinet.net.au
Website: www.dyslexia-speld.com

SPELD Queensland Inc
PO Box 2214
Milton BC 4064
Tel.: (07) 3262 9844
Email: speld@speld.org.au
Website: www.speld.org.au

CHAPTER AUTHOR

Paul R. Whiting
The Evelyn McCloughan Children's Centre
Faculty of Education
University of Sydney
64 Laurence St
Pennant Hills NSW 2120
Australia
Tel.: (61 2) 9875 1240
Email: whitingpr@yahoo.com.au

DYSLEXIA IN AUSTRIA

Maria Götzinger-Hiebner and Michael Kalmár

INTRODUCTION

Dyslexia, understood as an impairment of the acquisition of reading/writing/spelling in otherwise bright children, has been widely known and accepted in Austria since the 1950s, due to the work of Dr Lotte Schenk-Danzinger, the legendary 'Mother of Dyslexia'. (She cheerfully adopted this title and, in her late years, changed it herself into 'Grandmother'.) Dr Schenk-Danzinger was a psychologist and the mother of a dyslexic child, and worked on the scientific level as well as on the level of school practice. Her books on dyslexia are still standard literature in German-speaking countries. Together with Othmar Kowarik, a special needs teacher, she set up classes for dyslexic children and free training courses outwith school in Vienna, which ensured a high level of awareness and acceptance among teachers. In the 1980s, her concept was abandoned in favour of an all-embracing 'integrative multisensory' approach for children with different kinds of learning difficulties. In the past decade, dyslexia has become a topic again. Initiatives have sprung up in different parts of Austria – private groups such as Österreichischer Bundesverband Legasthenie, and groups of psychologists working in schools and universities.

LEGISLATION

In Austria, school legislation is centralized. Curricula are issued by the Federal Ministry of Education for all schools. However, regional boards of education (one for each of the nine federal states) can make their own interpretation and there is ample provision to do so. That means that, in fact, we have a federal situation granting the regional boards a high degree of autonomy. In the past few years, school authorities have begun to accept their responsibility for dyslexic children and students in primary and secondary schools. In a number of regulations, teachers are requested to consider the problems connected with dyslexia, especially in written exams.

International Book of Dyslexia: A Guide to Practice and Resources. Edited by Ian Smythe, John Everatt and Robin Salter. ISBN 0-471-49646-4. © 2004 John Wiley & Sons, Ltd.

TEACHER TRAINING

The teacher training institutes are generally free to determine their curricula. Some information on dyslexia is offered. Courses that give teachers more detailed information are rare, and usually not obligatory.

Advanced teacher training institutes are independent of the teacher training colleges. Their task is the post-graduate training of teachers. Some of them provide full courses on the treatment of dyslexia in schools. However, their curricula differ widely from each other. There is also a course offered by the University of Salzburg. Although the situation is improving, there is still a lack of qualified help in schools, and much is left to the private sector.

Illiteracy in adults is seen as a problem and some adult training centres provide instruction in reading, writing and maths. They are usually not aware that part of their clientele is dyslexic.

THE WORK OF NGOS

In 1991, the first national Austrian dyslexia organization – the Österreichischer Bundesverband Legasthenie – was founded by a group of parents, psychologists and teachers. Dr Lotte Schenk-Danzinger was a founding member and the association is still very much obliged to her.

The Bundesverband provides free counselling for parents and teachers in personal meetings and through a telephone help-line. The association does not offer assessment or therapy but helps parents to find qualified professionals if needed. It publishes a quarterly journal and information brochures. Among its other activities are lectures and workshops for teachers and parents and training courses for teachers and therapists, both in the private sector and in advanced teacher training institutes. A great deal of grass roots work is done to improve the situation.

A number of other (mostly regional) dyslexia organizations have since been founded. In 1998, a second national dyslexia association, the Erster Österreichischer Dachverband Legasthenie (EOEDL) was founded in Klagenfurt by the leaders of a regional organization. In cooperation with the Firstcybertrade Inc. and the Kärntner Landesverband Legasthenie, the EOEDL offers a distance learning course that leads to a diploma as a dyslexia trainer.

ORGANIZATIONS

Österreichischer Bundesverband Legasthenie
c/o Mag. Magda Klein-Strasser
Rosentalgasse 11/13
A-1140 Vienna
Tel.: +43 1/911 32 770
Fax: +43 1/911 32 777
Website: www.legasthenie.org
Email: info@legasthenie.org

Erster Österreichischer Dachverband Legasthenie
Feldmarschall Conrad-Platz 7
A-9020 Klagenfurt
Tel/fax: +43 463/556 60
Website: www.legasthenie.at

Arkus
Rechter Iselweg 5
A-9900 Lienz
Tel/fax: +43 4852/69822 or 64085
Email: arkus@gmx.at

Burgenländischer Landesverband Legasthenie
Tel.: +43 2682/64 2 44
Tel.: +43 664/56 50 896

Kärntner Landesverband Legasthenie
Feldmarschall Conrad-Platz 7
A-9020 Klagenfurt
Tel./fax: +43 463/556 60
Website: www.legasthenie.com

LEGA Vorarlberg
PO Box 201
A-6901 Bregenz
Tel.: +43 676/54 18 917
Tel.: +43 5574/74 888

Niederösterreichischer Landesverband Legasthenie
St. Poeltner Strasse 11
A-3233 Kilb
Tel.: +43 2748/7827

Oberösterreichischer Landesverband Legasthenie
Blütenstrae 23
PO Box 208
A-4041 Linz
Tel./fax: +43 732/71 12 83
Email: schulter.lentia@nvb.at

Salzburger Landesverband Legasthenie
Gislarweg 3
A-5300 Hallwang
Tel.: +43 662/662 180
Email: eva.roth@salzburg.co.at

Steirischer Landesverband Legasthenie
Mandellstraße 4
A-8010 Graz
Tel.: +43 316/82 95 60
Email: hposch_1@iaik.tu-graz.ac.at

Tiroler Landesverband Legasthenie
c/o Dr Heinz Zangerle
Tel.: +43 512/58 42 18

Wiener Landesverband Legasthenie
Wallgasse 26/17
A-1060 Vienna
Tel.: +43 1/913 38 53
Email: AW-versandservice@teleweb.at

CHAPTER AUTHORS

Mag. Maria Götzinger-Hiebner
Former President of the Österreichischer Bundesverband Legasthenie, Member of the Board

Michael Kalmár
Board Member of the Österreichischer Bundesverband Legasthenie, second Vice-President of the Board of the European Dyslexia Association

DYSLEXIA IN BAHRAIN

Haya Al-Mannai

INTRODUCTION

In the State of Bahrain, research development in the field of dyslexia is still in its infancy and at first sight it might even appear to be relatively ignored. But this paradox requires closer scrutiny, as we begin to examine the meaning behind the word 'dyslexia', as it is understood here in Bahrain.

It will be made clearer that this problem has been addressed earlier under various terms such as 'learning difficulty' or 'Arabic language disability' as opposed to the actual word 'dyslexia'. It is only when we realize this particular situation that a better understanding of the problem is revealed.

To begin with, the Ministry of Education supervises all aspects of education in the State of Bahrain and the small size of Bahrain has helped in achieving this educational 'centrality'. Formal education is free to all children and schooling is compulsory at the elementary and intermediate levels. Consequently, a child with a learning difficulty would be more likely to receive free support only at the primary level of schooling. Continued support in either 'Mathematics' or 'Arabic Language' at the elementary level is not available.

Moreover, pre-school screening depends largely on whether or not the child attends kindergarten and if experienced teachers are available to examine those children suffering from learning disabilities. Help and support would then depend on the parents' financial situation and their awareness of the importance of early intervention. Even then, to find appropriate, specialized local help is not easy.

THE ROLE OF THE MINISTRY OF EDUCATION IN 'SPECIAL EDUCATION'

In 1986, the Ministry of Education began showing an interest in a group of learning disabled students and formed a Special Education Committee for the primary level of edu-

International Book of Dyslexia: A Guide to Practice and Resources. Edited by Ian Smythe, John Everatt and Robin Salter. ISBN 0-471-49646-4. © 2004 John Wiley & Sons, Ltd.

cation. This was led by the Assistant Under-Secretary for General and Technical Education, Mr Hasan Al-Muhri. It included experts from all parts of the country who had worked in this field. The efforts of the Special Education Committee were supported and guided by the College of Education of the Arabian Gulf University. Its College of Education focuses on special education and offers diplomas and master's certificates in either 'Mental Retardation' and 'Learning Disability' or the 'Education of the Gifted and Talented'.

The year 1986 was a turning point for the group of disabled learners. The Special Education Committee made efforts to retrain certain distinguished teachers by sending them for a diploma qualification in the Special Education programme at the Arabian Gulf University. The Special Education division began with just three teachers having only a diploma qualification in special education, and presently it has 39 qualified teachers with a postgraduate qualification (diploma or master's) from the Arabian Gulf University.

Currently, out of about 114 primary government schools, 63 government schools (approximately 55 per cent), have a teacher specialized in the area of learning difficulties. The size of the school determines whether the teacher will be posted there on a permanent or temporary basis. The larger the school, the more likely it is for a Special Education teacher to be stationed permanently in it.

Diagnosis of students with mental and/or physical handicap and disabled learners begins upon entry into the school. Three evaluations are taken to determine whether a student is suffering from any difficulties: (1) results of student achievement in classrooms; (2) that of the class teacher; and (3) the diagnosis of the Special Education teacher. If all three evaluations suggest a student is having difficulty, an effort is then made to help the student.

Mentally and/or physically handicapped students are sent to the Medical Psychiatry division at the Salmaniya Hospital for further diagnosis. At this point, according to the student's level of handicap, they are transferred to another government institution that caters for his or her disability. Such institutions are the Saudi-Bahraini Institute for the Welfare of the Blind, the Al-Amal Institute and the Social Rehabilitation Centre.

However, with regard to the group of disabled learners, they are kept in their own school but are given special help in their particular areas of difficulties. Usually, the help is provided in the subjects of Arabic Language or Mathematics.

With the co-operation of the Arabian Gulf University, the Special Education divisions at the Ministry of Education were able to develop what they called the 'Academic Diagnostic Assessment Tests' for Arabic Language and Mathematics. The former subject is made up of three levels and the latter is composed of six levels. Through continuously reviewing the group of disabled learners, these diagnostic tools have been standardized four times from 1986 to the present.

SUPPORT FROM THE SPECIAL EDUCATION UNIT

Support for those students who are learning disabled is offered individually and takes two forms. The first involves receiving training in the academic skills they find difficult from a special education teacher in a special resource room. This one-to-one tutorial is temporary and is offered in only one of the two subjects of either Arabic Language or Mathematics in which the student is having difficulty. For the remaining subjects the student is returned to the normal classroom to join the other students. Once a disabled learner shows improvement in the particular area of difficulty, they are returned to the regular schooling schedule of the classroom.

The criteria used to determine a disabled learner's improvement are the student's school achievement results. If the student fulfils the minimum 'Adequacy Requirements' for the grade level that has been set by the Directorate of Curriculum Education, then this is an indication of improvement.

The second form of support to the disabled learner is offered indirectly. Here the special education teacher advises the classroom teacher on appropriate ways of dealing with the student who has undergone the special care treatment.

The remedial support system has its advantages and disadvantages. Some of the advantages are as follows. This system is a flexible way of offering students support during different times of the year. Also, it is economical because it caters for a large number of students who appear to require additional academic support and it prevents that group of disabled learners from being completely separated from their peers. On the other hand, the disadvantages of this support system appear during and after the remedial programme. One of the disadvantages during the remedial programme is that those individuals under treatment may feel inferior in relation to their peers, particularly in those subjects closely related to their learning disability.

With regard to disadvantages that follow the remedial programme, some are of concern to classroom teachers who are constrained by factors, such as time, which prevent them from offering the student the most effective and continuous support. Moreover, the lack of awareness of some of the parents of students suffering from a 'language' or a 'mathematical' disability implies that the only help they receive is during the short period they have with the special education teacher.

Also, lack of support from parents could be because one or both of the parents are of non-Arabic origin and hence do not speak the language at home, thus widening the gap for their disabled learner. According to the Educational Statistics (Information and Documentation Centre, 1995/96) published by the Ministry of Education, there are about 19 known nationalities enrolled in primary education in Bahrain. Three of those are of non-Arabic origin, e.g. Indians, Pakistanis and Iranian. They comprise approximately 2 per cent of the total student population enrolled in primary education and approximately 26 per cent of the total non-Bahrain elementary student population.

BRIEF ANALYSIS OF MA STUDIES IN THE LEARNING DIFFICULTY AREA

The earliest MA study in the area of learning difficulties that was carried out in Bahrain was at the Arabian Gulf University in 1995. Since then to date an estimated 20 postgraduate studies have been carried out at the same university. Of them, 55 per cent of MA research work was carried out in Bahrain, 30 per cent in Kuwait, 5 per cent in Saudi Arabia and 10 per cent in Qatar.

From among the studies that have been carried out in Bahrain, nine studies were on reading difficulties. Five of these studies used a descriptive approach in their research and four studies used the experimental approach. From among the former research approach, two studies looked into the relationship between reading and memory, two studies looked into the relationship between reading difficulty and social skills, and one study examined the relationship between reading difficulties and perceptual skills.

However, with regard to the latter approach (i.e. the experimental approach), the studies on reading difficulties mostly involved assessing the effectiveness of a certain teaching strategy or a remedial programme in improving performance in a particular reading area among subjects diagnosed to have language difficulty.

THE ROLE OF THE UNIVERSITY OF BAHRAIN REGARDING THE TOPIC OF LEARNING DIFFICULTIES

The University of Bahrain has only recently become interested in the topic of learning difficulties. One of the earliest signs of interest in this topic appeared in March 1998, when the Department of Psychology held a three-day workshop entitled 'Assessment and Teaching of Dyslexic Children' led by Dr Michael Thomson of East Court School for dyslexic children in England. The workshop was attended by participants representing the Ministry of Education, the Ministry of Labour, the BDF Hospital, the College of Health and Science, the Al-Amal Institute for Handicapped Children, the Psychology Department as well as five private schools.

As a response to the workshop, the Psychology Department, which is part of the University of Bahrain's College of Education, received many phone calls from parents asking for help with their children, and this can be regarded as one of the prime motivators in encouraging the Psychology Department to introduce the BA programme 'Educational Psychology of Special Groups'.

There are no local societies or private educational associations dedicated to children with learning difficulties.

FUTURE OUTLOOK

So far, the Ministry of Education, which is solely responsible for all educational matters in the country, has been the main party involved in handling learning problems such as dyslexia among students. This central control of the educational process has been seen to be advantageous in enabling the progress of education among the 'normal' population and making it available to everybody.

Unfortunately, progress has been relatively slower for those students whose learning difficulties stem from a psychological disability than for those students suffering from a mental and physical disability. Hence, the absence of an apparent physical disability among the former group of students may have made their identification difficult and may have contributed to the slow progress in the learning difficulty areas, e.g. dyslexia.

People will be able to see that these students are not scholastic failures but simply require a different way of teaching unlike other 'normal' students. Moreover, by being taught in specialized institutions, students with learning difficulty will be free from any comparison with regular grading systems administered to 'normal' students and will be allowed to progress at their own pace.

To conclude, it is hoped that this brief chapter will help shed some light on this important matter for all those concerned in order to gain a clear picture of this learning difficulty problem within the culture and structure of the Arabic language.

REFERENCES

Al Muhri, H. (1986) *Wakeah Al Idara AlTrbawiya fi Al Bahrain.* [The Position of Educational Administration in Bahrain.] State of Bahrain: Ministry of Education.

Arabian Gulf University pamphlet *Ba'd Ashir Sanawat min Nokta't Al-Bidayah, 1395–1405 Hijri, 1975–1985 Miladi.* [After Ten Years from the Starting Point, 1975–1985] Bahrain: Information and Cultural Relations, Arabian Gulf University.

Hummud, R.S. (1987) *Ata'lim fi Al-Bahrain.* [Education in Bahrain.] Riyadh, Saudi Arabia: The Arab Bureau of Education for the Gulf States.

Information and Documentation Centre (1995) *Educational Statistics 1995/96.* The State of Bahrain: Ministry of Education, Educational Statistics Section.

Kamal, A. (1994) *Al Suobat Al Marifyiah Wistratygiyat Al Tashkis Walmualijh.* [Cognitive Difficulties and the Strategies of Diagnosis and Remedy.] State of Bahrain: Ministry of Education, Directorate of Primary Education.

Ministry of Education (1986) *Ministry Decree No. 86/6/1025,* Ministry of Education Legislation and Disciplinary Directory. The State of Bahrain: Ministry of Education.

Urayid, F.A. (2000) Wagi'h Al-Tarbiyah Al-Kasah fi Al-Bahrain bayi'n 1980–1998. [The position of special education in Bahrain between 1980–1998.] *Al-Tarbyia* [*Education*, The Ministry of Education Educational Journal, Bahrain], No. 1.

Zuhair, A. (2000) Reaiyat Thawi AlIhtiajat Alkahsa Bil Madaris AlIbtidaeya Bi Dawlat AlBahrain. [Caring for Special Educational Group in the Elementary Schools of Bahrain.] Paper presented at a seminar in local and Gulf societies on Disabled Care between Reality and Ambition, Directorate of Primary Education, State of Bahrain.

ORGANIZATIONS

Directorate of Primary Education
Ministry of Education
The State of Bahrain

Arabian Gulf University
The State of Bahrain

Psychology Department
College of Education
University of Bahrain

CHAPTER AUTHOR

Haya Al-Mannai
Instructor
Psychology Department
University of Bahrain
PO Box 32038
Sakhir
Bahrain
Email: hayaalmannai@yahoo.co.uk

DYSLEXIA IN BELGIUM

Eleni Grammaticos and Anny Cooreman

INTRODUCTION

In Belgium, dyslexia, also referred to as specific learning difficulties, affects up to 5 per cent of the school population. Belgium has a unique situation since the country is run in three different official languages: French, Flemish, and German. In this chapter, Eleni Grammaticos discusses the situation from the French perspective, as well as the common aspects, while Anny Cooreman adds information specifically about the Dutch perspective.

PROFESSIONAL AWARENESS OF DYSLEXIA

In the past two years Belgium has improved as far as the professional awareness of dyslexia is concerned. TV programmes have been shown and books, brochures and articles have been published and have focused on dyslexia prevention and early recognition. With the help of the French government, brochures (including *Dyslexie, où est la différence?* written by M. Klees and E. Grammaticos) have been freely distributed to all teachers working in the French part of the country and dealing with 5-year-old to 7-year-old children. This specific brochure deals with early recognition, assessment, solution and treatment.

The non-governmental organization VZW Die-'s-lekti-kus, with the support of Cera Foundation and the Belgian government, has helped develop professional awareness of dyslexia among teachers, school administrators and parents in the Dutch-speaking community. In 2001 a first aid kit with a video entitled 'Don't call me stupid', and a CD-ROM were developed and offered free to all Dutch-speaking schools for all age groups. Since October 2002 a website www.letop.be has made it possible for parents and teachers to find: an agenda for most activities about dyslexia and other learning disabilities; a forum to exchange ideas; and a large library with easy-to-read articles with many ideas that can be put into practice.

International Book of Dyslexia: A Guide to Practice and Resources. Edited by Ian Smythe, John Everatt and Robin Salter. ISBN 0-471-49646-4. © 2004 John Wiley & Sons, Ltd.

As a consequence of these and other activities, many schools are now aware of the need for specific support for children with learning disabilities. Primary schools have more training in handling these problems than secondary schools. But both still have a lot of work to do.

WHO CAN ASSESS THE CHILD WITH SPECIFIC LEARNING DIFFICULTIES?

In Belgium there are centres operating independently from schools (but closely collaborating with them) which play an important role from pre-school to the end of secondary education in assessment, counselling, and educational guidance. In these centres, called psycho-medical-social centres (or *centres PMS* in French or *CLB* in Dutch), the child is assessed by an educational psychologist, who will try to give an objective view of the child's abilities and difficulties and then specify recommendations for remedial help. Medical check-ups are also included, and are important for the overall assessment of a child with dyslexia. The aim of such a check-up is to eliminate other causes that can have similar effects. Parents are usually advised to arrange sight, hearing, or other medical check-ups, as well as a neurological examination.

The assessment can also be administered by a Guidance Centre (*Centre de Guidance* for French-speaking children and the *Revalidatiecentra* for Dutch-speaking children), in which case the child is evaluated by an interdisciplinary team which includes an educational psychologist and also a speech and language therapist (*logopède/logopedist*). Here again, the aim of the assessment will be to highlight the child's abilities and difficulties. A qualified speech therapist may also carry out assessment and remedial work. One can also choose to be tested at a local university hospital, where rehabilitation services can be provided and advice given. In all cases there is a long waiting list.

REMEDIAL WORK

After the assessment, if this is necessary, the child will be offered a course of educational therapy. Remedial work is carried out by speech therapists, working in schools, in hospitals, or in private practice, or coming to the child's home. Parents can choose the speech therapist they want, which is usually the one nearest to them. Educational help takes place usually one or two times a week and is state-reimbursed for at least two years. It is also possible to look for a learning disabilities specialist. However, there are few lists of addresses available, so sometimes it can be difficult to find the remedial help your child needs. The Revalidatiecentra can offer remedial teaching, but children have to be severely impaired and need help for three different problems at the same time.

COST OF REMEDIATION

On the one hand, remedial sessions can either be free (or nearly free, meaning that the patient must pay a very small part of the total amount) or not. To benefit from (nearly) free remedial sessions, parents must go to *centres PMS* or *CLB*, to the *Centre de Guidance/Revalidatiecentra*, or to a university hospital, which are very good centres. On the other hand, if a patient goes to a speech therapist, for instance, they will have to pay for the rehabilitation help but will be partially reimbursed by the Belgian Health Care System (called *Mutuelle/Ziekenkas*). As a guide, one can expect to pay about 31 Euros per hour for individual rehabilitation sessions. The *Mutuelle/Ziekenkas* will reimburse around two-thirds of this amount, and sometimes more.

Reimbursement, for the rehabilitation of dyslexic difficulties, will be given to parents for a period of at least two years. After that period, it is usually more difficult to benefit longer from state reimbursement even if the child still needs help, and the parents will have to pay the total amount.

SPECIAL EDUCATIONAL NEEDS AND LEGISLATION

In the Belgian system, special assistance for children who are unable to learn satisfactorily in the normal classroom is in the hands of a series of specialized schools. Schools are subdivided into eight categories. The disabilities handled by these schools range from children with specific learning difficulties to the severely mentally handicapped and retarded. Schools intended for children with specific learning difficulties are identified under the label 'Type 8'. Before the child can join any special education courses, he or she must be assessed by a centre or by therapists (psychologists, speech therapists) working in hospitals, and receive a medical certificate of admission. These Type 8 schools are public and free.

In ordinary schools, the classroom teacher is not trained enough to recognize and deal with learning difficulties and to adapt their teaching methods to different learning styles. Some special training is offered to teachers, either during their studies or afterwards when they start work, but it remains difficult for them to help children with severe specific learning difficulties because there are too many children in a classroom (around 25, or even more).

The aim of Type 8 schools is to help children overcome their difficulties, to fill the gaps, to encourage and develop the child's capabilities, as well as to rebuild their self-confidence. In short, the aim is to reintegrate the child, as soon as possible and in the best conditions, into ordinary schools.

The advantages of Type 8 schools are numerous: there are few students in a classroom; classroom teachers know a lot about learning difficulties and adapt their teaching methods; each child can work at their own rate. Speech therapy and the help of psychometricians are included in the educational schedule and are free.

Unfortunately, there are also disadvantages and an important one is that Type 8 schools do not exist beyond elementary school. So that even if a child with specific learning difficulties were to continue as a Type 8 child in the secondary school, they are obliged to reintegrate into ordinary schools.

WHAT CAN WE DO TO IMPROVE THE SITUATION?

Associations and professionals are fighting for the right of children with learning difficulties, for teachers and parents to have access to information and advisors, to training programmes, and to appropriate help. Although dyslexia is recognized in Belgium and different and specific help is offered, we should continue to fight to improve the rights of all dyslexic children. Examples may include:

- give the child the right to pass oral exams instead of written ones;
- give the child more time to read and answer a question during a test or an exam;
- give the dyslexic child texts instead of making them copy from the blackboard;
- exempt, if necessary, the dyslexic child from learning other languages;
- support the work of teachers dealing with dyslexia as well as parents;
- offer day or evening classes for adult dyslexics;
- extend the period of reimbursement (two years of rehabilitation as a minimum);
- give the dyslexic child the possibility to continue as a Type 8 in the secondary school;
- let the dyslexic child use a laptop at an early stage.

REFERENCES

Cooreman, A. and Bringmans, M. (2002) *'Ik heet niet dom' Leren leven met leerstoornissen*, Leuven: Acco.

'Eerste Hulp bij Leerstoornissen' Die-'s-lekti-kus (2001), www. letop.be

Klees, M. and Grammaticos, E. (2000) *Dyslexie, où est la différence?* 2nd edition. IPEJ asbl. Jacques Layry, rue Falise 37, 1470 Baisy-Thy, Belgium.

ORGANIZATIONS

APEDA (Association de Parents d'Enfants en Difficulté d'Apprentissage)
Av. du Prince Héritier 10
1200 Bruxelles
Belgium
Tel./Fax: +32 2 763 33 78
Email: fmm.turbhall@belgacom.net

Vzw Die-'s-lekti-kus
Diestsesteenweg 722
3010 Kessel-Lo
Belgium
Fax: 016 35 64 32
Email: info@dieslektikus.be
Website: www.letop.be

CHAPTER AUTHORS

French
Eleni Grammaticos
President of APEDA
Neurolinguist
Erasme Hospital
Neuropediatric Department
808 route de Lennik
1070 Bruxelles
Belgium
Email: Eleni.grammaticos@ulb.ac.be

Dutch
Anny Cooreman
Vice-President of Vzw Die-'s-lekti-kus
Email: info@dieslektikus.be

DYSLEXIA IN BRAZIL

Ian Smythe

INTRODUCTION

Brazil is the largest country in South America, with a population of 173 million (2000) in a country of 8.5 million square kilometres (slightly smaller than the USA). The Brazilian population is over 80 per cent urban, and there is a very distinct economic divide. The top 5 per cent of the population control well over 50 per cent of the national economy. The main language spoken in Brazil is Brazilian Portuguese, with significant amounts of German, Polish, Spanish, Dutch, Italian and Japanese, as well as indigenous languages spoken in rural areas. An estimated 32 per cent of the rural population lives below the poverty line, and the top 20 per cent of the population controls 63 per cent of the nation's wealth. Officially adult illiteracy is 15 per cent, but while 97 per cent of the population enrol in primary school, only 66 per cent attend secondary school.

POLICIES AND LEGISLATION

In the early 1990s there was a reorganization of the government departments, and the Secretariat for Special Education became part of the National Secretariat for Basic Education as a Coordinating Board for the Supplementary and Special Education Department of the Ministry of Education. As a consequence, the importance of special education diminished, and several ongoing projects, including those with international bodies, were stopped.

New legislation (Law no. 8.490), introduced in November 1992, improved the situation with the creation of the Special Education Secretariat within the framework of the Ministry of Education, which has led to improved funding and resources. Programmes, including vocational training for the disabled, were started to help individuals with all types of special needs.

Following wide consultation, the first National Special Educational policy was instituted in 1994, and still provides the principal guidelines for progress in this sector.

International Book of Dyslexia: A Guide to Practice and Resources. Edited by Ian Smythe, John Everatt and Robin Salter. ISBN 0-471-49646-4. © 2004 John Wiley & Sons, Ltd.

Implementation followed, and led to the development of the Law of Basic Guidelines in 1996, which set out the principles for inclusive education for all SEN individuals in Brazil, including those suffering from dyslexia, deficits in attention and hyperactivity. Although the government clearly indicates its desire to incorporate the guideline principle in education by stating that it has achieved this in almost half of the 5,000 municipalities, there is some concern that a lack of understanding, a lack of resources, and sometimes a resistance to change, have meant that in some cases the result has been integration rather than inclusion. That is, the individual is made to fit into the system, rather than the system being modified to ensure it can cater for the diversity of children with special education needs. Examples include failure to provide appropriate resources and facilities. Furthermore, unlike recent legislation in other countries, this does not include the need for an educational plan or suggest the need for parental participation in the educational process. In November 2001, the Law of Inclusive Education (Law no. 10.172) came into effect, which means that from now on dyslexic students cannot be turned down by any Brazilian school.

Although not a participant in the Salamanca Conference, and therefore not an original signatory to the Salamanca Declaration, Brazilian clear intent has been shown through, for example, the development of the National Curricular Parameters which demonstrate at least a desire to respect individual differences. In the wider context of SEN, there is obvious commitment to the policies. However, while, for example, television programmes have been broadcast on the use of information technology with the SEN child, this has tended to concentrate on those with physical difficulties, including motor difficulties, as well as the deaf and blind communities. There is little indication of, say, programmes about using software, or how to use technology with the learning disabled. This is so, not only because there is no software to support such programmes, but also there are no individuals seeking to develop this area of expertise in Brazil.

In 1998, through its Curricular Adaptations, the government defined a strategy for helping students with special needs and attempted to create a climate within the educational system of 'Education in Diversity'. This included improving teacher training programmes and increasing involvement with teacher training professionals.

The rhetoric of government policies suggests there is an interest in developing educational practice in the direction laid out in the Salamanca Declaration. That is, there is an attempt to do the following:

- to recognize a need to take full account of individual differences (Statement 21);
- to adapt to the needs of the child (Statement 28);
- to provide additional assistance and support to children requiring it (Statement 29);
- to identify difficulties and assist pupils to overcome them (Statement 31);
- to provide appropriate teacher training (Statement 42).

TEACHER TRAINING

Despite an increasing amount of quality research which could inform teaching practice, there is almost no mention of specific learning difficulties within teacher training. This may be seen as a reflection of the level of understanding within all sectors. There are two sides to this: first, there is nobody at government policy level who has sufficient understanding of the issues to decree that it should be part of the teacher training curriculum and, second, there are few people who could develop such a curriculum. If operating in a local context, they have certainly not offered it widely. Consequently, training and class-room support for these children are, at best, highly fragmented.

IMPLICATIONS

It has been noted that while there are special needs policies in place, none refer to learning disabilities, and there is no legislation that ensures the school will implement a proposal to improve an individual's situation. Therefore, the conclusions are that the legislation does not do the following and should do so:

- support teacher training in learning disabilities;
- require the schools to provide assessment procedures;
- provide guidelines on the assessment and review process;
- explicitly state the need for differentiation and allow for individual difference, other than in the most general sense.

It is felt that until such time as there is greater parent power, which develops through knowledge and understanding of the difficulties, the legislation is unlikely to change. As that parent power increases, so the demands for fair education and legal challenges to the failure to provide appropriate education will increase, particularly with the 'duty of care' that is currently in place in other areas such as the medical profession. If the government fails to move in the desired direction, there will no doubt be court cases brought, whereby the pockets of good practice will provide the evidence for the need for, and viability of, change.

RECOGNITION IN SCHOOLS

While legislation mentions special education needs, there is no requirement on the part of the school to carry out a formal assessment procedure. This is entirely at the discretion of the school. Teachers do not receive any formal training in either the identification or remediation of children with learning disabilities. Therefore, these children are only recognized after considerable failure at school. Once a difficulty has been acknowledged, the parents can either wait up to six months for a free state-provided assessment, or pay for a private assessment, assuming, that is, that they are in one of the major cities where that assessment is available.

There are many individuals who may become involved with the diagnosis of dyslexia, and it is not uncommon for a child to be transferred from one professional to another to identify the specific difficulties. These professionals may include psychologists, neuro-linguists, speech and language therapists, paediatricians and even psychiatrists, each of whom will charge a fee for their services.

There are no standardized tests in Portuguese that would identify learning disability or the underlying cognitive difficulties. Despite research demonstrating the ease of producing simple, informative tests (see, for example, Capovilla and Capovilla, 2000; Capovilla et al., 2001), no standard measures are yet available. Each professional will use their own battery of tests and questionnaires, which are often more about the designation of a label with respect to an external (English language-based) criterion, as opposed to the use of assessment tools which would inform the individual education plan and teaching practice.

Use of the Weschler Intelligence Scale for Children is not uncommon, sometimes as part of a discrepancy-based diagnosis, and sometimes as a useful source of some of the standardized subtests (e.g. digit span). Assessment reports are usually minimal, with a confirmation of difficulties rather than an extensive list of specific difficulties, and what to do about them.

There are few centres which specialize in dyslexia assessment. In São Paulo, the largest is the ABD centre. In Rio de Janeiro there are several clinics, the largest of which is that of Paulo Mattos MD at the Centro de Neuropsicologia Aplicada. There is another large clinic at Maringa in the south of the country.

TEACHING RESOURCES

One of the key issues concerning dyslexia is that the whole area of reading in Brazil appears to be built on false premises (see Capovilla and Capovilla, 2000). The Portuguese language is fairly regular, and as such is ideally suited to a phonics-based programme. However, the current policy is based on a whole-word approach. It has been suggested that implementation of a phonics programme would not only help the learning disabled child, but also improve the rate of acquisition of literacy skills in all children. These resources are generally not available in schools.

ADVOCACY GROUPS

Associação Brasileria de Dislexia (ABD)

This organization was formed in 1981, and has a membership concentrated in the São Paulo area. They run teacher training courses, and, thanks to early commercial support (Grupo Fenica), they have established headquarters, complete with conference rooms, library, etc. Though originally set up by a parent as an information centre, it now also has a Reference Centre for assessments and teachers' courses. The organization has also been involved in the development of a television programme on dyslexia, but this is only available pay-to-view television.

Associação National de Dislexia (AND)

The Associação National de Dislexia (AND) was established in 2000 to provide dyslexia support in the region of Rio de Janeiro, as well as other parts of the country. The organization held its first conference in November 2001, having been officially formed earlier that year. Overwhelming interest has led to the production of its first training course, which started in April 2002. Other activities include an assessment centre (including bursaries for those on a low income) and a website which carries valuable information.

Associação de Dislexia de Rio Grande de Sol

The Associação de Dislexia de Rio Grande de Sol is an academic-based organization started in November 2000, attempting to serve the south of Brazil. They have a small website, but appear not to be particularly web-literate as demonstrated by having a 427,000 byte logo on their front page!

ACKNOWLEDGEMENTS

Ian Smythe has been to Brazil on a number of occasions, speaks fluent Portuguese and has carried out research in Brazil. He would like to acknowledge the contributions of Carla Moita and Alessandra Capovilla in writing this chapter.

REFERENCES

Capovilla, A.G.S. and Capovilla, F.C. (2000) *Problemas de leitura e escrita: Como identificar, prevenir e remediar numa abordagem fônica.* São Paulo, SP: Memnon-FAPESP.
Capovilla, A., Smythe, I., Capovilla, F. and Everatt, J. (2001) Adaptação brasileira do International Dyslexia Test: Perfil cognitivo de crianças com escrita pobre. *Temas sobre Desenvolvimento,* 10, 30–37.

ORGANIZATIONS

Speech and language therapy services
Website: br.cade.dir.yahoo.com/compras_e_servicos/saude/Fonoaudiologia/

Associação Brasileira do Déficit de Atenção (ABDA)
Website: www.dda.med.br/assoc01.shtml

Associação Brasileira de Dislexia
Website: www.dislexia.org.br/oquee.html

Associação Nacional de Dislexia
Website: www.andislexia.org.br/

Centro de Informação sobre Dislexia
Website: www.wdnf.info/brasil

Associação de Dislexia de Rio Grande de Sol
Website: http://ad-rs.vilabol.uol.com.br/

CHAPTER AUTHOR

Ian Smythe
34 Collingwood Road
Sutton
Surrey, SM1 2RZ
United Kingdom
Tel.: +44 20 8770 0888
Email: ian.smythe@ukonline.co.uk

DYSLEXIA IN BULGARIA

Vanya Matanova

THE SCHOOL SYSTEM IN BULGARIA

The Bulgarian school system has two stages: primary (basic) (divided into primary and pre-gymnasium) and secondary (high). The primary school provides education for 7- to 11-year-old children. The pre-gymnasium covers up to 14-year-old children, and the secondary education is up to 19 years of age.

Bulgarian is the official language. Bulgarians comprise the major ethnic group in Bulgaria. There are also other ethnic groups, the largest of which are Turkish and Gypsy (Roma) groups. The Turks live in compact communities in certain regions of Bulgaria and communicate among themselves in Turkish, but the school education is conducted in Bulgarian. Recently, teaching of the Turkish language on a voluntary basis has been provided at schools in the areas inhabited by Turks.

Gypsies live in compact groups spread all over Bulgaria. The majority of them are not covered by the school net. A considerable proportion of formal education Gypsies drop out of by the end of primary school. They speak Gypsy dialects among themselves but are taught in Bulgarian. The Gypsy dialects have only oral versions. The Gypsies in general live in very poor environments since the majority of them are unemployed. For a variety of reasons, many Gypsy children attend special schools for the mentally retarded, which are maintained by the government.

LEGISLATION AND POLICIES

All children in Bulgaria have the right to education embodied in the Constitution and the National Enlightenment Law. According to the Law for Protection of the Disabled, every child with identified disabilities has the right to receive special support in relevant special schools.

The activities of the logopaedical units are fixed in the decrees of the Ministry of National Enlightenment. According to them, children with reading and writing difficulties

International Book of Dyslexia: A Guide to Practice and Resources. Edited by Ian Smythe, John Everatt and Robin Salter. ISBN 0-471-49646-4. © 2004 John Wiley & Sons, Ltd.

are eligible for this special service. These children attend mainstream schools and receive special support in the units for speech and language therapy.

DEFINITION AND TERMINOLOGY

Under the influence of the Russian 'defectological' school, in Bulgaria the terms 'dyslexia' and 'dysgraphia' have for a long time served to indicate difficulties in reading and writing, respectively. In the past decade, however, the term 'specific learning difficulties' has become more popular. There is still a debate between specialists whether the terms 'dyslexia' and 'specific learning disabilities' are completely equivalent. Nevertheless, the majority of professionals adopt the following definition:

> Dyslexia is a summative group of disabilities caused by disintegration of perceptual, cognitive and language abilities, that influences the ways of input, elaboration and storage of linguistic type of information, which manifests itself by difficulties in acquiring the basic school skills – reading, writing and maths. These disabilities are not related to mental retardation, sensory impairments, severe emotional disturbances or behavioural disorders, nor to social, or cultural factors.

IDENTIFICATION AND ASSESSMENT

The process of identification of problems in acquiring basic school skills, i.e. reading, writing and maths, usually takes place in second or third grade. Identification is based upon the teacher's perceptions of failures in following the school curriculum. Early predictors of dyslexia are looked for in relation to language deficits in pre-school years.

Various kinds of specialists are responsible for identification and assessment, including psychologists, speech therapists, child neurologists, child psychiatrists, etc. The speech therapists are those who deal with the intense assessment that involves determination of the development level of high cortex functions, as well as of reading and writing skills. The psychological assessment focuses on measuring the current intellectual functioning, specifics of the cognitive processes, self-esteem, self-image, etc. Unfortunately, those cases diagnosed as dyslexia are not a matter of team discussions and thus the particular specialists diagnose and treat only their separate parts of this multifaceted phenomenon.

INTERVENTION AND RESOURCES

The intervention is provided primarily by speech therapists in mainstream schools. The children receive additional extra-curricular support. The duration of a session at the speech therapist's centre is about 45 minutes and takes place two to three times a week. The therapeutic support concerns writing disturbances. In Sofia (the capital of Bulgaria with a population of about 2,000,000), there are about 40 centres of this kind. Such intervention organization precludes teamwork and thus certain deficits remain hidden.

TEACHER TRAINING

The discipline of Psychology is taught at five Bulgarian universities (three state and two private), while the discipline of Special Education (which currently covers Speech and

Language Pathology and Therapy) is established in eight universities. These two disciplines deal with the issues of dyslexia. The students become familiar with the basic characteristics, diagnostic criteria, and therapeutic approaches to dyslexia in the frame of the module 'Abnormal Psychology', which constitutes a part of the curriculum in Psychology.

The speciality of Speech and Language Pathology and Therapy provides considerably wider and more thorough knowledge of the field of dyslexia. The discipline to cover all these issues is usually formulated as 'Writing Disorders in Specific Learning Disabilities'.

Unfortunately, students in the specialities of Primary and Pre-school Education are not provided with any kind of knowledge related to dyslexia. This ultimately explains one of the reasons why dyslexia is sometimes identified so late.

Until now, there have been two PhD theses and two monographs on the issues of dyslexia in Bulgaria. These are 'Disturbances in Reading and Writing' by Ivan Kerekovski and 'Dyslexia' by Vanya Matanova. Many Bulgarian and foreign articles concerning the issues of dyslexia have been published in the specialized periodicals in medicine, psychology and education. In the past few years, seminars on dyslexia for mainstream teachers have been implemented.

ADVOCACY, VOLUNTARY AND PROFESSIONAL GROUPS

There is no national association on dyslexia in Bulgaria. In 2001, the Bulgarian Reading Association was set up; it deals with the development of prevention and intervention programmes in the field of dyslexia. In the same year, the Bulgarian Association for Logopaedics and Phoniatrics held a conference on the topic of dyslexia. There is no association for the parents of children with dyslexia.

EXAM AND CURRICULUM PROVISIONS

Children with dyslexia follow the mainstream school curriculum. It means that no alternative educational programmes exist with respect to literacy in particular. In some cases, students take oral exams, but most work and the admission exams to some kinds of schools are in written form, so children with dyslexia are at a disadvantage.

PROVISIONS FOR ADULTS

Support for adults with dyslexia takes place at medical institutions in cases of acquired alexia-dyslexia, occurring as a consequence of strokes and cerebral trauma.

THE WAY AHEAD

Future progress is directed towards:

• identification of early predictors of dyslexia so that prevention programmes can be developed;

- introduction of a compulsory screening test to be implemented before entering school;
- design of training courses for teachers to handle the instruction of dyslexic children;
- organization and popularization of team-work practice with respect to dyslexics;
- development and introduction of alternative programmes with respect to acquiring literacy;
- organization of mobile classes for students with dyslexia in mainstream schools.

CHAPTER AUTHOR

Vanya Matanova
Department of Social, Work and Educational Psychology
Sofia University
Tzar Osvoboditel 15
Sofia
Bulgaria
Email: v_matanova@yahoo.com

DYSLEXIA IN CANADA

Linda S. Siegel

INTRODUCTION

The term dyslexia is not widely used in Canada; it is not a popular term. The reason for this reluctance to use this terminology is not clear; it may be that the term 'dyslexia' was originally associated with the medical profession and it is generally believed that learning difficulties fall within the domain of educators and psychologists. Although 'a rose by any other name may still smell as sweet', quibbling over the name dyslexia is still a problem in the educational and psychological community.

What is called dyslexia in other countries is called a learning disability (LD) in Canada. A learning disability means that the individual (child or adult) has difficulty in one more academic area, such as reading, writing, spelling or arithmetic, but is of average or above average intelligence. What are called 'learning disabilities' in Canada are called 'learning difficulties' in other places. Dyslexia is not the only learning disability; there are problems with arithmetic, and/or mathematics that may also occur and these may be mistakenly called dyslexia. However, spelling and arithmetic/mathematics difficulties without the reading problems are of concern; they are not dyslexia which is a very severe reading problem (Siegel, 1999).

CANADA: BACKGROUND

Canada is a vast country with a relatively small but diverse population of approximately 27 million. The geographical extent of the country with a population spread out and often in relatively isolated areas poses special problems for children with learning disabilities. Present-day Canada has been characterized as a 'vertical mosaic' (Porter, 1965) in that it includes a unique mixture of several cultures. These cultures include the native peoples, or First Nations, who were the original inhabitants; Canadians of French descent, whose ancestors settled in Canada during the seventeenth and eighteenth centuries; Canadians of British descent, whose ancestors came to Canada from Britain from the seventeenth century onward; from the United States during the American Revolution in the latter part

International Book of Dyslexia: A Guide to Practice and Resources. Edited by Ian Smythe, John Everatt and Robin Salter. ISBN 0-471-49646-4. © 2004 John Wiley & Sons, Ltd.

of the eighteenth century, and immigrants from all over the world. Immigration occurred in three waves: in the latter part of the nineteenth century and early twentieth century, immigrants from Asia (mainly China) came to the west coast of Canada. Immigrants from various European countries came to central Canada and the prairie provinces during the early twentieth century and following World War II. More recently, Canada has received a large influx of immigrants and refugees, mostly from countries in economic or political turmoil in Latin America, the Caribbean, Asia, the Indian subcontinent, what was formerly the USSR, and the Middle East. All of these cultural groups have had a major influence on Canadian society and education, including the education of children with learning disabilities (Siegel and Wiener, 1993).

SOCIETAL AND CULTURAL FACTORS AFFECTING THE EDUCATION OF CHILDREN WITH LD

Five societal and cultural factors were identified as having an impact on the education received by children with learning disabilities in Canada. First, and perhaps overriding all other factors, is that education is exclusively a provincial jurisdiction in a federal political system. Consequently, legislation, policies, and procedures vary significantly from province to province. Second, official bilingualism has implications for students with learning disabilities who must either study or learn in a second language. Students with English as a first language are expected to learn French and vice versa. Third, in addition to the English- and French-speaking populations, Canada has a large multicultural community. The dominant Canadian ethos is that these communities should maintain the culture of their country of origin while simultaneously integrating into Canadian society. Differentiating learning disabilities from problems with English or French as a second or other language is a major diagnostic issue. Fourth, 1.3 per cent of children in Canada are from native communities and have specific language, learning, and cultural needs. Fifth, Canada has a relatively well-developed social safety net (i.e., provision of education, health, and social services through government funding), which has led to the expectation that services for children with learning disabilities would be provided, for the most part, by the public sector.

INCLUSION AS A POLICY

From the first recognition of learning disabilities in the late 1950s and early 1960s, the understanding has become increasingly sophisticated. Every Canadian province and territory recognizes the existence of learning disabilities. Most provinces have total inclusion of children with learning disabilities, or are moving rapidly toward that goal. That means that all children, whatever the disability, receive instruction in regular classes, although they may be withdrawn for special services. This policy can pose a special challenge for teachers who have students with learning disabilities in their classrooms.

CHALLENGES

I will highlight some recent recommendations that we made in a report to the British Columbia Ministry of Education (Siegel and Ladyman, 2000). These recommendations illustrate what has been accomplished in Canada and what needs further attention in the treatment of dyslexia and other learning disabilities.

Most educational systems in Canada have virtually total inclusion. There is, however, withdrawal with specialized teachers for children with learning disabilities. This inclusion is proceeding well and is generally successful but there are certain aspects that should be noted. Inclusion works best with smaller class sizes (20–25 is typical) and with appropriate support for the teacher. As many teachers were educated in an era when inclusion was not the norm, professional development and additional training are required for these teachers. Tuition fee rebates to help develop special education knowledge and an understanding of successful methods are a worthwhile goal but not, as yet, a reality. It is very important that special education be part of the general teacher education curriculum, with emphasis on specifically how to help children with various kinds of learning difficulties.

The geography of Canada poses special problems. Teachers and students are often in remote locations. A much greater exploration of distance education to help students in remote areas is needed.

Funding is typically provided on the basis of the disability. We distinguish between 'low incidence' condition such as blindness, deafness and physical handicaps and 'high incidence' or more commonly occurring difficulties in the incidence of learning disabilities in Canada. Learning disabilities fall into the high incidence category. However, there are no reliable demographic data. Although learning disabilities have typically been funded on a per child basis with intensive testing and identification required, we propose moving to a system where student skills are carefully monitored and the district receives money for special education proportional to the number of students enrolled in the system, rather than on the number of students specifically identified as special education students. However, it is important that the funding be targeted for special education. The system has the advantage of minimizing the assessment, reporting and auditing necessary to obtain special education for the student.

EARLY IDENTIFICATION AND INTERVENTION

The emphasis is moving towards early identification in intervention for learning disabilities. In a pilot programme in North Vancouver, British Columbia, kindergarten children were identified with an increased battery of language phonological awareness and memory tasks (Lesaux and Siegel, 2002). If found to be at risk, they were given a phonological awareness programme in the context of a balanced literacy programme. The children's progress was monitored at the end of each grade. As in many districts in Canada, there is a significant portion of children in this district who have English as a second language. When the children entered kindergarten, 40 per cent of the children had English as a second language or were considered to be at risk for reading difficulties and 25 per cent of the children had English as a first language or were considered to be at risk. At the end of Grade three, 3.5 per cent of the children who had English as a first language were found to have dyslexia and 2.5 per cent of the children with English as a second language were found to have a significant reading disability.

The challenges for individuals with learning disabilities are that different agencies are responsible for them at different periods of their lives. The Ministry of Education is only responsible for children in elementary and secondary education. Before that, it is the

Ministry of Social Services and the Ministry of Health. Unfortunately, records are not easily transferred from ministry to ministry and many children fall through the cracks. They may have had language, speech or motor difficulties identified before they enter school but this information does not reach the school. The transition to post-secondary education or employment is also difficult and, again, records are not transferred.

One of the major challenges for individuals with dyslexia and other learning disabilities is the provision of sufficient technology (software and computers) which is critical in helping them to compensate for their difficulties. Unfortunately, this technology is not always available in the quantity that it should be.

Individual education plans (IEPs) are a requirement in most jurisdictions in Canada. Often these are very successful but sometimes teachers have not received sufficient guidance in developing these IEPs. Parents are required to be invited to participate in the process but sometimes the process breaks down and sometimes the IEP may represent merely paperwork, not a systematic plan for the student. Clearly, more planning and development are needed to make the IEPs an important educational reality.

Students with a learning disability are allowed to take the provincial exams with more time and sometimes orally. However, there is still resentment of this process and resistance to it.

When students drop out of school or are suspended from school, it may be a result of untreated or undiagnosed learning disabilities. School violence may also be a consequence of learning disabilities that are not successfully recognized and remain untreated. Street youths are likely to have undiagnosed learning disabilities as are adolescents who commit suicide (Barwick and Siegel, 1996; McBride and Siegel, 1997). For this reason it is important to monitor the progress of all students in reading, spelling, arithmetic and writing.

Canada is moving in the direction of monitoring these skills in all students and recognizing that any difficulty may mean a learning disability that requires further investigation.

THE WAY AHEAD

Funding for special education is always insufficient and until the Canadian government recognizes this, it will be a problem. The best hope is early identification and early intervention. In addition, we must carefully monitor the reading, spelling, arithmetic, writing and mathematical problem skills of all students to ensure that all learning disabilities are recognized and that the children receive help for them.

REFERENCES

Barwick, M.A. and Siegel, L.S. (1996) Learning difficulties in adolescent clients of a shelter for runaway and homeless street youths. *Journal of Research on Adolescence*, 6, 649–670.

Lesaux, N. and Siegel, L.S. (2002) Preventing reading failure: Findings from a 5-year longitudinal study. Paper presented at International Academy for Research in Learning Disabilities, Washington, DC, June.

McBride, H. and Siegel, L.S. (1997) Learning disabilities and adolescent suicide. *Journal of Learning Disabilities*, 30, 652–659.

Porter, J. (1965) *The Vertical Mosaic: An Analysis of Social Class and Power in Canada*. Toronto: Carswell.

Siegel, L.S. (1999) Issues in the definition and diagnosis of learning disabilities: A perspective on *Guckenberger v. Boston University. Journal of Learning Disabilities*, 32, 304–319.

Siegel, L.S. and Ladyman, S. (2000) *Review of Special Education in British Columbia: Report for the Province of British Columbia*. British Columbia: Ministry of Education.

Siegel, L.S. and Wiener, J. (1993) Canadian special education policies: Children with learning disabilities in a bilingual and multicultural society. *Social Policy Report*, 7, 1–16.

ORGANIZATION

International Dyslexia Association
Website: www.interdys.org

CHAPTER AUTHOR

Linda Siegel
Educational and Counselling Psychology and Special Education
University of British Columbia
Faculty of Education
2125 Main Mall
Vancouver, BC V6T 1Z4
Tel: (604) 822-5513
Email: linda.siegel@ubc.ca

DYSLEXIA IN THE CARIBBEAN

Rosey Palmer

INTRODUCTION

Work in the area of dyslexia is of fairly recent origin in the Caribbean. Preoccupied, formerly, by the macro-task of developing a viable education system for global effectiveness, the territories of the region may have paid less attention to individual variations in learning than countries with long-established traditions of scholastic exposure, if not of inclusive provision. In the years surrounding the turn of the millennium, Jamaica, having established its high school programme (the Rose Curriculum) and having instituted the staged examination procedures which lead up to it through the primary years, the NAP tests including the Grade Four Reading Test and the GSAT, is now considering earnestly the needs of those who fall through the net. It is in this context that an initiative taken in the 1970s and contacts made in the mid-1990s have come together to stir an understanding of the difference which inhibits selective scholastic skills yet liberates the affected individual to the kind of achievements attained by Winston Churchill, Thomas Edison, Albert Einstein, Whoopi Goldberg and Garth Vaz.

This chapter seeks to trace the influences which have led Jamaica to the verge of a turnaround in education which will no longer consider the late reader as an unfortunate misfit in the educational system, but as a person with special potential who needs careful individualized nurturing.

HOW THE ADULT DYSLEXIA ORGANIZATION STARTED IN JAMAICA

In 1995 Owen Sinclair, a well-known businessman in the west of Jamaica, now Custos Rotolorum of Westmoreland, sent a group of young men to Mrs Rosey Palmer for tuition and thus initiated one of the most subtle and far-reaching developments in education in the west of Jamaica since the government's decision to provide education for all. Bearing many questions in mind as to why these young men had been unable to benefit from six years of primary education and the opportunity to spend three to five years in the

International Book of Dyslexia: A Guide to Practice and Resources. Edited by Ian Smythe, John Everatt and Robin Salter. ISBN 0-471-49646-4. © 2004 John Wiley & Sons, Ltd.

secondary classroom, Mrs Palmer attended Jamaica Expo'96 in London where she exhibited the developmental reading and writing work done at her preparatory school. The work attracted the attention of Selwyn Wright, then the Public Relations Officer of the Adult Dyslexic Association.

During an in-depth conversation about the disability, Mrs Palmer recognized the pattern of learning that Owen Sinclair had brought to her attention. Subsequently, for four years the skill of extending the reading ability, not only of young adults, but also of school students who were referred to DELA Children's Workshop for help was practised and shared. Selwyn Wright found time to visit, from England and help to establish a Westmoreland Dyslexia Organization for dyslexics and their families. In 1999 Barbara Stewart, of the Chamber of Commerce, observed that difficulties experienced by some trainees in the government's school leavers' employment orientation scheme had become a matter of concern among business people and a file containing information about dyslexia was prepared for the consideration of the Chamber of Commerce. Copies were also submitted to the Parish Library and to the Regional Office of the Ministry of Education and Culture.

Currently research work is being carried out in government schools in the parish to assess the feasibility of reading interventions for dyslexics within mainstream education. Although the condition is stressed in the Special Needs Programmes of the teachers colleges, groups are eager to support non-government sponsored seminars and workshops on the topic. Indeed, Mico Teachers College hosted the visit of the Caribbean Dyslexia Centre to Jamaica in June 2000.

THE STATUS OF DYSLEXIA AWARENESS IN JAMAICA

One of the major causes of 4 to 20 per cent of individual learning difficulties worldwide, dyslexia is known as the difference in mental functions which makes certain skills difficult to attain and to practise. Jamaican teachers have noticed specific difficulties in learning to write, learning to read, learning to spell, ordering, counting and mastering other mathematical procedures, organizing and orienting oneself and one's belongings. However, as dyslexia has not been widely diagnosed at the high school level, its association with average or high levels of general intelligence and particular creative and inventive abilities is often unsuspected. The losses about which researchers warn readers in the field of dyslexia, which, by marginalizing affected individuals, affect the capacity of a society to survive economically, are, doubtless, having their effect on the local scene. Although no wide-ranging assessment of the incidence of dyslexia in Jamaica has yet been carried out, its occurrence across the full socio-economic range and its recurrence in successive generations of the same families have been observed. Correlations have also been noted between unrecognized dyslexia, which often results in illiteracy, and incidence of criminalization.

Dyslexia was studied in Jamaica over 25 years ago by Dr Barbara Matalon in her seminal research into learning difficulties. At that time, the term dyslexia had not yet acquired the breadth of meaning that current worldwide research and publicity have given it, so, to avoid too narrow a focus, Dr Matalon referred to the related traits of the dyslexic student as specific learning difficulties. It is under this title that the work in Jamaica had progressed to the highly developed diagnostic and remediation procedures, available in some parts of the island. Now, as a result of the input of the Caribbean Dyslexia Centre and the efforts in the west of the island as outlined above, the condition is beginning to be known and understood in such a way that its full implications can be addressed.

SUPPORT FROM THE CARIBBEAN DYSLEXIA CENTRE IN BARBADOS

Background

The foundation of a specialist centre for dyslexia in Barbados stemmed from the concern of parents whose children were experiencing the condition and dedicated teachers who worked with them. It began with a partnership between Sylvia Johnson and Yvonne Spencer who, with Mary Crouch, called a public meeting in March 1994 to establish a project which was acknowledged by the Ministry of Education but has been funded through the faith of the participants. The venture has been resourced by the Hornsby International Dyslexia Centre in England, which sent a team of professionals, consisting of Professor Colin Terrel, Maria Farrer, and Joan Durr, to hold a one-day workshop with 55 interested people in Barbados in May 1994. This group pledged to start the centre which would, initially, be staffed from London and would offer a correspondence course for teaching dyslexic students as well as educational courses for affected persons. Through changes of personnel and venue, the centre has grown to assist over 325 students, 20 young adults and many teachers. Classes are now assisted by Maria Hutson, an Orton Dyslexia trained tutor, assisted by Marcia Farnham. Since 1999 a Caribbean-based Teaching Dyslexic Pupils Course, taught during the months of July and August annually, has been available at the centre. Parent support groups and talks to schools and other organizations are featured but, most significantly for the Caribbean, the centre has a regional outreach thrust.

Inter-island outreach

The brainchild of co-ordinator, Yvonne Spencer, this programme was funded by the Caribbean Development Bank and offered neighbouring countries one-week workshops on the awareness of dyslexia. The programme was spearheaded by Marilyn Monaghan and targeted 18 territories: St Lucia; Grenada; St Kitts; Nevis; the Bahamas; the British Virgin Islands; Montserrat; Anguilla; Dominica; St Vincent and Bequai, the Grenadines and Turks and Caicos, Jamaica and others. Overwhelming numbers of teachers and parents responded to the opportunity and benefited from sensitization to the concepts of dyslexia and its related conditions, diagnostic testing, cognitive profiling, multi-sensory teaching, and study skills. Sessions were both theoretical and practical and activities included observation of a specialist teacher at work with children who experience learning difficulties. Teachers were awarded a certificate for the course and parents had an opportunity to air their concerns and to create a support network with others whose children share common difficulties.

THE CURRENT SITUATION IN JAMAICA

Thus, Jamaica, as many other Caribbean territories, is now becoming aware of the need to diagnose the learning difficulties of under-achievers and to provide opportunities for remediation to those children who cannot be adequately served by standard pedagogic delivery. A 1999 summer course, mounted by a group of concerned parents for children with learning difficulties and their teachers, and the seminar mounted by the Caribbean Dyslexia Centre, Barbados, both had a lasting impact on public awareness.

The work of the Mico Care Centre is known countrywide and students who are referred there for diagnostic testing can attend invaluable part-time classes if they reside in the corporate area. Intervention in the homes of under-achieving students in other parishes is facilitated by the Private Volunteers Organization, which, for example, works with Sam Sharpe Teachers College in the west. Aid is also available from the Jamaica Association for Children with Learning Disabilities and Jamal. Both these facilities have their headquarters in Kingston, though Jamal has branches in the parishes.

The Adult Dyslexia Organization (ADO), based in Westmoreland, has been associated with a dyslexia unit formerly held at DELA Children's Workshop in Smithfield. However, under the presidency of Trevor Swaby, the ADO has as its main thrust the development of awareness among teachers in the government system. It offers input to parent–teacher meetings, to the media and to staff meetings and departmental meetings in conjunction with the Westmoreland Inter-Schools' Reading Association whose mission is to promote reading as a skill and a leisure activity to children of all ages. Within the scope of the ADO lies liaison not only with the Ministry of Education and Culture but also with National Security and Justice, in order to press for reading instruction in Jamaica's prisons. The brief of the organization extends to hosting international conferences, to adapt tests to the local language and culture, and to empower teachers to use them in the classroom to diagnose children with specific difficulties. This undertaking is in the context of the government's imperative: to ensure literacy for all school-leavers by the year 2003.

Westmoreland Inter-Schools' Reading Association (WISRA) was also able to provide another boost to public awareness of dyslexia when Dr Garth Vaz, a member of the Orton Society in America, arrived in the parish to launch the biography of his brother, A. McDonald Vaz, *The Doctor He Begged to Be*. These two dynamic ambassadors for special educational provision and assessment arrangements have spoken at a well-attended (WISRA) annual general meeting and at many other events around the island, pressing for medical, social and educational co-operation to address the challenges that face children who experience a broad spectrum of learning disabilities. The Jamaica Reading Association has been able to testify to the fact that special examination conditions have already been offered to affected students at Caribbean Examinations Certificate and at tertiary level in Jamaica and that the condition for such arrangements is diagnosis by a specialist teacher. Dr Vaz has introduced to Jamaica the broad-based testing which he practises in Texas by training Dr Ivan Rodriquez in the application of the tests. More public awareness is needed to benefit children who are now tested at Grade 4 level in a countrywide Reading Test administered by the Ministry of Education.

CONCLUSION

The message underlying the emerging focus on dyslexia in the Caribbean is an inspiring prospect not solely because of the students and families it stands to empower, but because of the mediation of the message through our own indigenous academia, the black diaspora in England, America and through our Caribbean neighbours. Caribbean educational research can be seen to have come of age when local participants in the arena find direction in the studies produced at the University of the West Indies. The family ties, in Jamaica, of founder members of the Adult Dyslexia Organization of Brixton, England, prompted them to respond vigorously to the need they discovered in their peers in Jamaica and enabled one of their number to follow up his interest in a timely and effective manner. The constant appeal of their birthplace has brought the Vaz brothers on many goodwill trips since their migration to the United States, yet the impact of their trip to launch *The Doctor He Begged to Be* is likely to be the most significant of all because they are confounding, by their undeniable success, the stereotypically negative response which the education system may have formerly entertained towards youngsters just like them. The vision of the Caribbean Dyslexia Centre and the sponsorship by the Caribbean Development Bank of their regional outreach programme implement an intra-territorial development plan which speaks of regional pro-active answers to the residual problems which were endemic to the historic colonial conflict. Discussions, which are annually reviewed at the Adult Dyslexia Organization conference, are expected to lead, not only to individual empowerment, but also to additional human resources for regional economic growth.

ORGANIZATIONS

Adult Dyslexia Organization, Jamaica
C/O The Secretary
Ms Virginia Turner Shrewsbury District Petersfield P.O. Petersfield
Westmoreland
Jamaica
Tel.: (1) 876 955 3011
Email: delawithrosey@yahoo.com

Note contact with Dr Rodriquez may be made through Mr Trevor Swaby on the above telephone number.

Caribbean Dyslexia Centre
Haggart Hall
St Michael
Barbados
Tel.: (246) 435 0387

Jamaica Association for Children with Learning Disabilities
7 Leinster Road
Kingston 5
Jamaica
Tel.: (1) 876 929 4341/4548

Mico Care Centre
5 Manhattan Road
Kingston 5
Jamaica
Tel.: (1) 876 754 5747

CHAPTER AUTHOR

Rosey Palmer
Lot 11 Smithfield
Savanna-la-Mar P.O.
Westmoreland
Jamaica
Email: delawithrosey@yahoo.com

DYSLEXIA IN CATALONIA

Dolors Juanola, Neus Buisán and Mercè Gonzàlez

INTRODUCTION

Catalonia is one of the autonomous regions within the Spanish state and has wide responsibilities in educational matters. There is not, however, sufficient recognition of dyslexia
in Catalonia or Spain. Dyslexics and their families often suffer the consequences of this
lack of information, found not only at the social level, but also in the school and health
systems. This lack is also widely acknowledged by the professionals who frequently show
a sincere interest in acquiring information about this matter, and who enthusiastically
attend the workshops that offer it.

Needless to say, this picture clearly defines the focus of the Catalan Dyslexia Association and its goal is as follows:

- to obtain full recognition of dyslexia from the authorities in education, health and
  employment;
- to organize activities that offer information to professionals in the field;
- to provide orientation to those affected by dyslexia and their families, to offer them
  support and to ease their anxiety by giving clear and precise information.

INFORMATION PROVIDED

In this chapter we would like to address a specific aspect of the information we offer to
the families that come to our association: how to face post-secondary education with possible success.

In Catalonia, the education system is organized as follows: three years of nursery school
(start at age 3), six of primary education, four of compulsory secondary education, and
two years of non-compulsory post-secondary education ('Batxillerat'). In the long road
from nursery school to the workplace, everybody, but especially dyslexics, has to endure
a battery of tests and trials and overcome several moments of crisis. Many of these

International Book of Dyslexia: A Guide to Practice and Resources. Edited by Ian Smythe, John Everatt and
Robin Salter. ISBN 0-471-49646-4. © 2004 John Wiley & Sons, Ltd.

moments occur when the teenage boy or girl has successfully completed compulsory secondary education and has to continue to the post-compulsory level.

Our association advises families to deal with the entrance to the post-secondary cycle in ample time, that is, to take action before the child finishes secondary school. The process begins by formally requesting the Catalan Department of Education Grants for a modification of the curriculum of 'Batxillerat' in the area of language and exemption from marking in the area of a foreign language (usually English). A 'curricular modification' is a licence the Department of Education may grant to some people who qualify for it. When it is granted, the department tells schools that the affected pupil is to be marked in these compulsory subjects, bearing in mind his or her personal characteristics. Although the student has to attend the lessons, do the homework, take tests and present papers, his or her spelling skills, for example, would not be marked by the usual standards. The interest in the modification of the area of language is especially important for our pupils, since they are required to present a full command of the two official languages of Catalonia: Catalan and Spanish.

DEALING WITH TWO LANGUAGES

What is the best way to proceed in the case of the foreign language requirement? It is true that at least at the written level, the foreign language usually poses an important problem for dyslexic pupils and that is why exemption of marking is requested in addition to the curriculum modifications. The student has to attend the lessons, but they will not be given a mark, so the mark in this subject will not affect their total point average, a factor which may be important in their entrance to university.

FURTHER EDUCATION

It seems obvious that the young pupil at this point in his or her academic career will have to overcome some reluctance. Should a person with this disability continue studying beyond compulsory education? Our society is undecided on this matter: some say, 'It is not necessary for everyone to study further', or 'university should be a place for excellence'. These and similar comments weigh heavily on our dyslexic students who are so used to struggling under unnecessary disadvantaged conditions. Without denying the previous statement, the Catalan Dyslexia Association defends the right of dyslexic people to study and to reach the highest levels. We claim that showing difficulty in certain aspects should not be a barrier to people's development, and this in no way implies that extraordinary results cannot be achieved in specific areas. Even now, this point has been amply proved by dyslexic people who are outstanding in their field, and many groups of people with physical handicaps have achieved recognition of their rights. Yet dyslexic people are still often advised against pursuing further studies.

CURRICULAR MODIFICATION

However, when should the curricular modification be requested? The entrance to the next educational stage should be prepared in the last year of compulsory education in order to have the curricular modification ready when post-compulsory studies begin. These documents cannot be improvised. The level of accuracy demanded by the education authorities is high and it is obviously in our best interest that it remains so. It is precisely because our purpose is to defend dyslexic people that we do not want this disability to be considered as some ineffectual disability affecting the population in general. We are therefore most concerned with obtaining a rigorous diagnostic. A diagnostic, nonetheless, which should not be too difficult to obtain from authorized public centres.

When the diagnosis has been obtained, the following documents should be compiled: first, a petition by the parents presenting their case requesting the modification and exemption from marking, and, second, a petition by the school for the same purpose. Documents from the inspector of the school district and from the teams of the school psychologist and educators are also useful, although these are difficult to obtain since there is still no official recognition of our cause.

The documents should be presented to the department who considers them, and will grant the curricular modification, specifying the affected subjects. Once the curriculum modification is communicated to the student and his or her family and to the school, aprocess begins for which there is little preparation at this stage. The directives of the department of education are of a general nature and the school has more and more autonomy to take decisions on this matter; however, it is often challenging for the teacher to know how to develop the specific details of the curricular modification on a day-to-day basis and here our association also offers orientation to the schools which may be a great help to them.

CONCLUSION

We should not accept a barrier that keeps our dyslexic students from achieving beyond compulsory secondary education. It is clear that they will not find much consensus nor help along the way. The Catalan Dyslexia Association is willing to move forward in this matter and both requests and needs the support of the people in our country but also of the European Union, who are often a reference point to us, and with whom we have to form a community without frontiers, to our mutual benefit.

ORGANIZATION

Catalan Dyslexia Association/Associació Catalana de Dislexia
C/Canet, 4
08017 Barcelona
Catalonia
Spain
Tel.: +34 93 203 03 46
Email: acd@infomail.lacaixa.es

CHAPTER AUTHORS

Dolors Juanola, Neus Buisán and Mercè Gonzàlez
Catalan Dyslexia Association
C/Canet, 4
08017 Barcelona
Catalonia
Spain

DYSLEXIA IN CHILE

Luis Bravo-Valdivieso

CHILE: BACKGROUND

Chile is a long and narrow country in the southwest of South America. Chilean people are a mixture of Spanish conqueror offspring, with other European immigrants and Indian original inhabitants. At present Chile has 14 million inhabitants who are split into a white middle-class minority, culturally and economically similar to the middle-class people belonging to other occidental countries, and a majority of lower-class people in culturally and economically deprived populations. They all speak Spanish. In Chile, between middle- and lower-class children there is a great cultural and economic gap. Low socio-economic status (SES) children show slower development in their cognitive and psycholinguistic abilities affecting their learning in the primary school and this brings about problems in reading and writing. About 5 per cent of them will become dyslexics. Among the low SES children there are many 'mixed' learning disabilities, with both neuropsychological and socio-cultural handicaps. Some researchers have shown that the psycholinguistic and phonological abilities of the low socio-economic children entering public schools are lower than those of children entering private middle-class schools (Bravo-Valdivieso, 1998).

Compulsory primary education started in 1920. At present it lasts eight years. Secondary education lasts four years and it is not compulsory. The school system is mixed, private and public. In the public system there are special schools for mentally retarded, blind and deaf children and 'differential pedagogical groups' for children with learning disabilities. Moreover, there are specialized teachers, trained at university, who help teachers on their courses to cope with children with learning difficulties (LD). Since 1974, children with LD can be sent to Diagnostic Centres, where they are diagnosed and enter differential groups without leaving their school.

In Chile there is a high prevalence of Reading Retardation (RR) and among schoolchildren who have been sent to the public Diagnostic Centres, the Reading Retardation srate is around 78 per cent. Most of these children belong to low SES schools (Bermeosolo

International Book of Dyslexia: A Guide to Practice and Resources. Edited by Ian Smythe, John Everatt and Robin Salter. ISBN 0-471-49646-4. © 2004 John Wiley & Sons, Ltd.

and Pinto, 1996). Moreover, some follow-up studies show that their prognosis in learning to read is poor and the initial reading retardation has a serious influence on the following school years (Bravo-Valdivieso, 1998).

The first studies in dyslexia were published in the 1960s and they were motivated principally by the high rate of holdover and drop-out among the children in the public schools. Most of these children failed in the primary school because of difficulties in learning to read and write.

In Chile, dyslexia is commonly defined as a 'severe and persistent reading retardation', in normal sensory and psychomotor children without mental retardation, independent of socio-economic status. Frequently, 'dyslexia' and 'severe reading retardation' are used interchangeably.

The early Chilean research in dyslexia was clinical, and originated in Neurological and Psychiatric Services for children. These studies describe the neuropsychological disabilities presented by reading retardation children as originating in a brain dysfunction. At that time, Olea and Moyano (1962) published an article regarding clinical research on dyslexic children. They associated dyslexia with a minimal brain dysfunction, that brought about deficits in visual perception, spatial orientation, and psychomotor development. Olea (1979) made a test for diagnosing dyslexia in children and to evaluate the integrity of the basic brain processing for learning to read. Following a neuropsychological perspective, Condemarín and Blomquist (1970) elaborated a test (TEDE) for assessing the initial reading and dyslexic problems in first grade children (Berdicewski et al., 1977). In 1973 Bravo-Valdivieso published a book including a neuro-psychological study done on a group of children who had been diagnosed as having 'minimal brain dysfunction'. The main difficulties of those children were related to learning to read and to write and therefore they were considered dyslexic. This research showed that they presented deficits in the development of their higher cognitive processes, such as the organization of thinking, reasoning and abstraction, as well as in perceptual and psychomotor abilities, that have disturbed their learning to read.

RESEARCH ON READING DISABILITIES AND SOCIO-ECONOMIC STATUS

The research on reading retardation and on dyslexia in children from low socio-economic status (SES) presents some methodological problems that are important for the Chilean research. Most of those low SES children have been handicapped by environmental deficiencies that can be the cause of their difficulties in reading and writing. Therefore, it is difficult for the researchers to distinguish in the samples children with reading retardation that is a consequence of their disadvantageous socio-economic background from children with dyslexia brought about by neuro-psychological, phonological developmental anomalies.

On the other hand, the known definition of dyslexia proposed by the World Federation of Neurology says that dyslexia can be diagnosed in the presence of socio-cultural opportunity, that is to say, disregarding the socio-cultural under-development of deprivation (Critchley, 1970). Therefore it precludes children from low SES being considered dyslexic. One consequence of this definition for researchers in the developing countries is that they could not include in their samples the majority of children from deprived socio-cultural environments. Nevertheless, to exclude socially disadvantaged children from research on learning disabilities and dyslexia is hardly realistic in a Latin American context. It would be particularly difficult to consider reading retarded children with low SES, as a category for exclusion, because poverty appears to be a permanent influence on school learning for the majority of them. Their socio-cultural variables should be taken into account in the research. One way to cope with the methodological problems derived from studying dyslexia among low SES children has been to compare matched groups of low SES children with severe Reading Retardation and normal readers who belong to the same schools and same social environments, where they receive similar environmental influences, and to follow them up.

A research study was done in a follow-up study during four school years with two groups of Chilean children who came from similar low-income families and schools. The aim of this research was to look for some neuropsychological and cognitive variables that discriminate between two groups from low socio-economic levels: one group of children who learned to read normally and another control group of severely reading retarded schoolmates. Both groups were equivalent in chronological age, grade, gender, IQ and SES (Bravo-Valdivieso, 1995).

The study showed that the greatest difference between them were in tasks of phonological awareness, in memory of visual sequenced letters for blending a word, in auditory comprehension of a story, and in verbal abstraction. These results confirmed that social deprivation did not appear to be the main cause of their reading disabilities. Moreover, in spite of their cultural and economic differences, the neuropsychological characteristics of this group of severely reading-retarded, low SES children appeared very similar to those found in more developed countries, when reading retardation and dyslexics are compared with normal readers. This research encouraged us to go on studying dyslexics among low SES children.

Another research study was done in Chile comparing severely reading retarded children belonging to two different socio-economic levels. A group of children with RR and another with normal reading (NR), from the middle and low socio-economic classes, were compared with the WISC R sub-tests. The aim of this research was to assess whether the neuropsychological differences between severe RR and normal reader children in each SES group were the same in both. Children belonging to both RR groups did not show significant difference in Verbal WISC IQ (Bravo-Valdivieso et al., 1991).

Results showed that the neuropsychological and cognitive WISC R sub-tests that discriminated between RR and NR in the low and middle SES groups were not the same. In the middle SES group, the RR children showed a worse performance in Similarities, Arithmetic, Blocks and Coding sub-tests. But in the low SES groups the significant differences between RR and NR children appeared in Sequences, Digit Span and Picture Completion. A two-year follow-up study of these groups showed that the low SES RR children persisted in having lower performance in these same sub-tests and in reading comprehension than control groups. This study allowed the conclusion that severe RR in low SES children is associated with lesser development in short-term memory and in visual-verbal-motor associations. The middle SES RR children instead showed difficulties in some higher cognitive and verbal processes. That is why, perhaps, they reach different levels in reading comprehension. Low SES children, normal and reading retarded, can have a more concrete and surface reading, and middle SES children can have a more abstract level in it.

PUBLIC AWARENESS AND TEACHER TRAINING

In 1968 several articles were published in the press, referring to the high cost of school failure, the numbers of those held back and the drop-out rate in public schools, caused by learning disabilities. Those articles made the educational authorities aware of the social problems brought about by the high rate of learning disabilities in the schools. As a consequence, the Catholic University of Chile created in 1969 the first graduate programmes for training teachers about learning disabilities and dyslexic children and to investigate this problem. Afterwards several other universities began to train teachers in special education for learning disabilities and dyslexias were included as topics in training primary school teachers.

In 1974 a group of psychologists and special education teachers belonging to five Chilean universities supported a national conference on special education run jointly with the Ministry of Education. At this conference the creation of a National Special Education system was proposed. This system was aimed to teach LD and dyslexic children in their schools. Special education was defined as 'a differentiated and interdisciplinary specialization of regular education addressed to those children who, whether due to transitory or permanent causes, are prevented from following the regular educational programme.' It was stated that special education must not constitute a segregated system apart from the general primary education and that its principal objective is to reincorporate the child, as quickly as possible, into the educational mainstream. 'The effectiveness of special education can be seriously compromised if it has to receive an overpopulation of children due to inadequacies in the regular education system.' They concluded by stating that work in special education must be complemented by preventative pre-school education. Therefore LD and dyslexic children are taught in differentiated groups within their schools, for several hours per week, following their normal courses during the rest of the day.

As far back as 1979 dyslexic children were taught according to a visual perspective and psychomotor models of dyslexia. In that year in Santiago, an international symposium of learning disabilities, sponsored by UNICEF, was held in the Catholic University, attended by Vellutino and Goodman. As a consequence, Chilean teachers and psychologists began to apply a verbal model for diagnosing and teaching dyslexic children. To assess RR and dyslexia some of the original tests of reading such as the TEDE are used (Berdicewski *et al.*, 1977).

In 1985, first in Chile and later in Spain, a book was published about dyslexia in Spanish-speaking children, and another in Mexico about language and dyslexia (Bravo-Valdivieso, 1985, 1988).

PRESENT TRENDS

Present trends in research in Chile have two objectives: (1) to assess the initial level of pre-reading and emergent reading in pre-school and first grade children; and (2) to determine some variables that could predict the achievement in reading in low SES children, during the primary school years. These have been financed by the Chilean Fund for Scientific Research (FONDECYT) and by the Catholic University (DIPUC).

REFERENCES

Berdicewski, O., Milicic, N. and Orellana, E. (1983) *Elaboración de Normas para la Prueba de Dislexia Específica de Condemarín-Blomquist*. Santiago de Chile: Universidad Catolica.

Berdicewski, O. *et al.* (1977) *Report for the Faculty of Education*. Santiago de Chile: Catholic University of Chile.

Bermeosolo, J. and Pinto, A. (1996) Caracterización de una muestra de alumnos asistentes a Group Diferencial. *Boletín de Investigacíon Educacional*, 11, 369–392.

Bravo-Valdivieso, L. (1973) *Trastorno del aprendizaje y de la conducta escolar*. Santiago de Chile: Edit. Nueva Universidad.

Bravo-Valdivieso, L. (1985) *Dislexias y retraso lector: Enfoque neuropsicológica*. Madrid: Ed Santillana.

Bravo-Valdivieso, L. (1998) *Lenguaje y dislexias*. Mexico: Ed Alfa Omega.

Bravo-Valdivieso, L. (1995) A four year follow-up study of low socioeconomic status Latin American children with reading difficulties. *International Journal of Disability, Development and Education*, 42, 189–202.

Bravo-Valdivieso, L., Berneosolo, J. and Pinto, A. (1991) Diferencias neuropsicológicas en niños con retardo en comprensión lectora de distintos niveles socioeconómicos. Paper presented to the IV National Congress of Psychologists, Santiago de Chile, August 1991.

Condemarín, M. and Blomquist, M. (1970) *La Dislexia: Manual de lectura correctiva*. Santiago: Edit. Universitaria.

Critchley, M. (1970) *The Dyslexic Child*. London: Charles Thomas.

Olea, R. (1979) Batería de integración cerebral funtional básica. *El Niño Limitado*, Special issue.

Olea, R. and Moyano, H.S. (1962) Acerca de las bases neurológicas de la dislexia de evolución. *Fonoaudiología*, 8, 22–24.

CHAPTER AUTHOR

Luis Bravo-Valdivieso
School of Psychology and the Faculty of Education
Catholic University of Chile
Santiago de Chile
Casilla 114-D
Santiago de Chile
Email: abravov@puc.cl

Dyslexia in China

Xiangzhi Meng and Xiaolin Zhou

THE CHINESE WRITING SYSTEM

The Chinese language is best known for its logographic writing system. In such a system, the basic orthographic units, the characters, correspond directly to morphemic meanings and to syllables in the spoken language. With some exceptions, each character represents one morpheme and has one pronunciation in isolation, although different characters may have the same or similar pronunciations. Because the number of syllables used in the language is limited to about 1,300, whereas the number of commonly used morphemes is about 5,000, Mandarin Chinese has a great many homophonic morphemes in the spoken and written language and many homophonic characters in the written language.

Unlike words in alphabetic scripts, Chinese characters have no direct grapheme–phoneme correspondences. However, it is worth noting that over 80 per cent of modern Chinese characters are so-called phonetic–semantic compounds. These characters consist of a phonetic radical part, which gives information on the pronunciation of the character, and a semantic radical part, which gives information concerning the meaning of the character.

RESEARCH

There is only a short history of research on developmental dyslexia in mainland China. Since the late 1990s, researchers in several psychological and medical departments of universities, such as Peking University and Beijing Normal University, have investigated the prevalence of dyslexia in Mandarin-speaking schoolchildren and the characteristics of their lexical processing.

It was found that 4–8 per cent of schoolchildren are dyslexic. Developmental dyslexics showed a larger phonological regularity effect in character naming and they rely more on the phonological code to access the semantic part than normal children. This indicates that lexical processing of Chinese characters is generally less efficient in developmental

International Book of Dyslexia: A Guide to Practice and Resources. Edited by Ian Smythe, John Everatt and Robin Salter. ISBN 0-471-49646-4. © 2004 John Wiley & Sons, Ltd.

dyslexics. They are confused on the use of the correct homophonic characters and they showed longer naming latencies in reading numbers and naming pictures as well as in reading characters. Cases of phonological dyslexia have been reported. The role of basic visual perceptual processing in reading development and dyslexia has also been investigated by the research group at Peking University.

It should be noted that most of the studies are carried out in Beijing, where school-children have a consistent Mandarin-speaking language background in schools and at home. But dialects exist in many other parts of China, which means that children speak dialects at home but read books in Mandarin at school. An interesting issue is then the impact of dialects on the development and manifestations of dyslexia in such children.

PRACTICE

There are many dyslexic children brought by their anxious parents to our laboratory and other institutes for help. Most of these children come from classes of medium and high grades. Their severe reading and writing difficulties make them underachieve not only in Chinese, but also in other subjects. Some of these children have behavioural problems as well.

In Beijing, besides our laboratory, there are several other centres providing help for children with learning difficulty. These centres routinely assess these children in many different cognitive domains, such as intelligence, memory, visual and auditory processing, balance, and other neurological tests. Their training programmes include sensory integration and visual and auditory drills. Programmes specializing in reading and writing training are rare, although such programmes are being developed in our laboratory.

To our dismay, there are still no standardized reading and writing tests for developmental dyslexia screening in mainland China, although vocabulary tests and other types of reading test have been developed but are not standardized in different laboratories and training centres. Results between different studies are not easy to compare.

ORGANIZATIONS

Although there are learning disability associations in mainland China, no societies are devoted to developmental dyslexia. However, due to the publication of books and articles in newspapers, parents and teachers in big cities are gradually accepting the concept of 'reading disability', even though in small cities and the countryside things largely remain the same. A specialized society for developmental dyslexia is being planned.

CHAPTER AUTHORS

Xiangzhi Meng and Xiaolin Zhou
Laboratory of Developmental Psychology
Department of Psychology
Peking University
Beijing 100871
China
Email: Mengxzh@pku.edu.cn

DYSLEXIA IN CROATIA

Nada Lovrić

PUBLIC AWARENESS

Pressure from parents of dyslexic children has been an important factor in stimulating public awareness of dyslexia in Croatia. Such pressure has led to the initiation of a number of activities that aim to protect the rights of dyslexics. A key reference book (such as the 1966 publication of *Reading and Writing Difficulties in School*, by Ribić and Matanović, a psychologist and a pedagogist respectively) and meetings (such as the 1972 Symposium on Dyslexia and Dysgraphia held in Zagreb, and the 1972 Congress of School Medicine held in Trogir) have further increased public and professional awareness of dyslexia by drawing attention to the existence of such disorders among children and adults. Additional pressure from parents of affected children has continued to encourage schools and other professionals, though their efforts have not always been successful and only occasional articles appear in the popular press. The Croatian Dyslexia Association (HUD), in co-operation with the European Dyslexia Association (EDA), provides a focus for the activities of parents and professionals. HUD publishes a twice-yearly bulletin and provides materials for teachers and parents who request it. Furthermore, representatives of HUD and activities organized by the association often appear on TV and radio.

PROFESSIONAL AWARENESS

In different regions of Croatia there are many professionals interested in developing a systematic approach to dyslexia and dysgraphia. The largest group of professionals involved in the diagnosis and remediation of dyslexic children are the logopaedists. The majority of these professionals work in Health Centres, though they are increasingly working in schools as well. Although the small number of psychologists engaged in schools means that further work is necessary to fully standardize diagnostic procedures, clinical psy-

International Book of Dyslexia: A Guide to Practice and Resources. Edited by Ian Smythe, John Everatt and Robin Salter. ISBN 0-471-49646-4. © 2004 John Wiley & Sons, Ltd.

chologists working in Health Service Centres have developed a detailed neuropsychological and psycholinguistic approach to the diagnosis of dyslexia and dysgraphia which can be used to inform remediation and school arrangements. Doctors specializing in school medicine screen for signs of dyslexia when assessing children's readiness for school, as do psychologists and logopaedists during the last year of kindergarten.

A positive feature is the increasing number of schools organizing seminars about dyslexia for teachers of primary classes. These one- to three-day seminars allow teachers to acquire basic knowledge of the area as well as to experience practice work. Members of HUD are co-ordinating such work with the Ministry of Education.

LEGISLATION

Children attend kindergarten from the age of three. It is a requirement (Education Law 1990) that children are screened for any signs of dyslexia at kindergarten level in order to prevent dyslexia-related problems damaging the child's development. Speech therapy and pre-reading/writing exercises are performed at the age of five and a half or earlier. However, these procedures are still not implemented in all towns and villages.

Children begin school at the age of six or earlier. A team of specialists (the Commission) must see each child as part of the Regulations of Entrance. Again, assessment procedures are performed to investigate possible signs of dyslexia as part of the process of determining readiness for school. If signs of dyslexia are evident, it is recommended that the child be observed at the school for three months (Educational Law 13/1991), after which a school team is required to produce a report about the child's progress that makes recommendations on further educational procedures. When signs of specific difficulties in reading, writing, spelling and/or numeracy are noted (by teachers, parents or specialists), a full diagnosis, detailing recommendations for remedial work and mode of schooling (see section on Assessment), is performed by a team of specialists. A final document is produced by the Town Department of the Ministry of Education and sent to the school and parents of the assessed child (Education Law NN 59/90, 27/93, 57/98). Dyslexia is included in Education Law NN 23/1991 as a specific learning disorder under item 3: Disorders of Communication of Speech and Language, Reading and Writing, Dyslexia, Alexia, Dysgraphia, Agraphia, Dyscalculia, Acalculia.

After primary-level education, there are few formal procedures. Although regulations exist for secondary schools (Education Law NN 19/92), very few, if any, dyslexics are diagnosed in secondary schools and there are too few specialists available to implement specific support procedures for such secondary-level children. Similarly, although the Centre for Professional Orientation takes account of specific difficulties, such as those experienced by dyslexic individuals, there are no provisions for job training. Finally, data about modifications at university level are not available.

ASSESSMENT

Screening for dyslexia is performed at pre-school age, both in kindergarten and when entering elementary school. However, the information obtained from these screening procedures is not always made available to schools. Even when it is forwarded to schools, most teachers are not trained in the specific needs of the dyslexic child and are therefore (at least initially) unable to provide appropriate support.

The most frequently used assessment procedure at school level is the One Minute Test (Furlan, 1965). When used appropriately, it can provide an initial insight into difficulties. An example of a less often used diagnostic procedure is the Test of Difficulties in Reading and Writing (Hadžiselimović). The International Test of Dyslexia (Smythe) is in the process of being translated and could provide further important information.

Once assessed as dyslexic, the child may be transferred to a specialist institution or centre. However, waiting lists for such specialist places are very long. When dyslexia is diagnosed, the child has the right (Education Law NN 23/91) to regular schooling with full integration. This may be based upon a regular curriculum, or one with certain adaptations through individual procedures and special help if available, or on a shortened programme with constant specialist support. However, only some 30 per cent of schools have the resources to implement the ideal procedure. Individual parents may be given advice and seek help outside of the school, although this may be a time-consuming process. The result is that many children are left without appropriate support.

REMEDIATION

One method of remediation comprises the Verbotonal Method (Guberina, 1985) with SUVAG Lingua (an electronic feedback device). In this procedure, incorrect auditory images of words are broken down and replaced by correct ones, leading to better speech habits and better concentration. In addition, the Pictographic Rhythmic method (Lovrić, 1984) is used as a multisensory approach to reading and writing (used mainly in the Polyclinic SUVAG, Zagreb). There are also a number of programmes involving pre-reading, pre-writing and writing exercises that have been developed by individual therapists in private centres or institutions, schools, Health Centres, etc.

The application of such techniques is most effective when conducted by teachers in the classroom with the assistance of a specialist in the method. However, there is a lack of funds and organization to purchase tools such as SUVAG Lingua equipment and provide professional assistance to teachers. Therefore remediation for the majority of children who receive it occurs outside of school. Also many experienced speech therapists and psychologists have been forced into retirement by the problems of the post-war economy and, hence, are not able to transfer their knowledge to the next generation of specialists. Waiting lists are growing with reductions in trained staff. It can now take three months for a diagnosis, with only one logopaedist (speech and language therapist) for three schools.

TEACHER TRAINING

Since 1996, there have been various efforts to create systematic training procedures for teachers. However, a lack of funds and political support has led to the majority of training events being confined to one- to three-day seminars organized by dedicated volunteers. The latest effort to improve this unworkable situation was a project (The Programme of Early Prevention of Dyslexia and Dysgraphia: Permanent Education of Pre-School Teachers, School Teachers and other School Specialists) proposed by HUD in 1999 and involving a group of psychologists and the Ministry of Education. Again, the lack of funds and the lack of sponsors have led to the project not being realized as yet.

REFERENCES

Furlan, I. (1965) *Jednominutni ispit glasnog čitanja.* Zagreb: Školska knjiga.
Guberina, P. and Gospodnetić, J. (1985) *Slušanje i govor u svjetlu Verbotonalne metode.* Zagreb: Centar SUVAG.
Guberina, P. and Pansini, M. (1985) *The Effects of the Spacioceptive Stimuli on the Intelligibility of Speech.* Project for Office of Special Education and Rehabilitative Services. US Department of Education, Washington, DC, and Zagreb: SUVAG.
Hadžiselimović, D. (1984) *Otkrivanje poremećaja u čitanju.* Zagreb: Školska knjiga.
Lovrić, M. (1984) *Metodika rada piktografske ritmike.* Zagreb: Centar SUVAG.
Lovrić, M. (1985) Pictographic rhythmics in the rehabilitation of hearing and speech of children with multiple disorders according to the principle of the Verbotonal method. *Zbornik radova III. Medunarodnog simpozija Verbotonalnog sistema.* Zagret: Centar SUVAG.
Novak Reiss, A. (1972) 'Zadaci školskog liječnika u problematici zaštite duševnog zdravlja školske djece i omladine'. *Zbornik radova I. kongresa liječnika školske medicine Hrvatske.* Zagreb: Informator.
Ribić, K. and Matanović, M. (1966) *Teškoće čitanja i pisanja u školi.* Zagreb: Školska knjiga.

ORGANIZATIONS

Hrvatska udruga za disleksiju (Croatian Dyslexia Association)
Kušlanova 59a
10000 Zagreb
Croatia
Fax: 1385 1 229 950
Email: lencek@antun.erf.hr

Polyclinic SUVAG for Rehabilitation of Hearing and Speech
Ljudevita Posavskog 10
10000 Zagreb
Croatia
Fax: +385 1 46 55166
Email: zagreb@suvag.hr

The Institute of Public Health
mr.sc. Juhović Markus V.
Mirogojska cesta 16
10000 Zagreb
Croatia
Fax: +385 1 62 17799
Email: vesna.markus@publichealth-zagreb.hr

CHAPTER AUTHOR

Nada Lovrić
Ivanieva 16
10000 Zagreb
Croatia
Email: maja.lovric@vip.hr

DYSLEXIA IN CYPRUS

Costas Apostolides

INTRODUCTION

In 1993 Cyprus had no policy on dyslexia in any area, though the approach to the subject was somewhat better in the Ministry of Health than in the Ministry of Education. The education system had legal provisions only for two special needs groups: the blind and the deaf. There was no comprehensive policy for children with special needs, and no educational policy other than a school for the blind, one for the deaf and three special needs primary schools.

Furthermore, few people in the Ministry of Education had heard of dyslexia, fewer still understood it, and some influential psychologists did not (and still do not) accept that it exists or that dyslexia has a scientific basis. There were no provisions for dyslexic children in the educational system, no special provisions for examinations, and the state education evaluation system was over-stretched. Furthermore, only two of the nine educational psychologists in the Ministry had sufficient knowledge to deal with dyslexia, while others did not even accept its existence.

The situation in the private sector was somewhat better, with a few qualified psychologists leading the way, and the main thrust being taken up by speech therapists who had training related to remediation of dyslexia, but who also did most of the diagnosis, owing to their greater experience than psychologists and special education specialists. Some private schools were also more willing to offer assistance to dyslexic children, but their intake was minimal because of entrance examinations.

The bureaucratic environment in the Ministry of Education was either indifferent or negative, with the exception of a handful of teachers, some of whom had training in special education. In general, the situation was better in the primary schools, which maintain a more pedagogic approach than the secondary schools.

Even more disturbing was the ignorance of the population at large, which resulted in most dyslexic children receiving no sympathy and being branded as lazy or indifferent to

International Book of Dyslexia: A Guide to Practice and Resources. Edited by Ian Smythe, John Everatt and Robin Salter. ISBN 0-471-49646-4. © 2004 John Wiley & Sons, Ltd.

learning, and with parents confused and not knowing where to turn for assistance. The main problems, however, were (and still are) with the lower income groups, who, in general, are faced with desperate problems.

PROGRESS WITH DYSLEXIA

The University of Cyprus in 1992, which had a strong department for training primary school teachers and included courses on special education including dyslexia, led to an improvement in the situation. This resulted in the new young teachers having at least an understanding of what dyslexia was, and since then this has influenced attitudes and improved the situation in the primary school system.

In 1993 the Cyprus Dyslexia Association (CDA) was established and registered as an association in January 1994. The objectives of the association in its rules and regulations were as follows:

- to help persons of all ages who have the dyslexia disability to develop their educational, cultural and other capabilities;
- to enlighten the public and the authorities with respect to dyslexia;
- to encourage officials to establish a state policy on dyslexia;
- to provide assistance to all the communities irrespective of religion or racial group or community, and to foreign residents of Cyprus;
- to create a centre for diagnosis, remediation and research.

The key factor here is that from the beginning the CDA had as one of its objectives the creation of a national policy on dyslexia.

Initially the emphasis was on providing information and educating both the public and officials as well as obtaining the support and guidance of the few private and state sector specialists that were active in diagnosis and remedial training. Its first acts were to publish a small pamphlet explaining what dyslexia is, organizing lectures, presentations and panel discussions and attracting media attention. The press, radio and television quickly reacted because they found that the public response was extraordinary, and was measurable through telephone requests for information from viewers and readers, who recognized that this could be the reason for the poor school performance of their children.

Providing guidance to parents and dyslexics took up most of the time of the association, but the capabilities for diagnosis and remediation were limited and still are. One problem is the acute lack of qualified specialists, though the situation is improving.

One of the initial weaknesses was the lack of information on dyslexia in Cyprus and this was overcome in part by CDA membership of the European Dyslexia Association and the International (American) Dyslexia Association, and co-operation and use of materials from the British and Greek associations.

PRIORITIES

The priorities for policy development as determined by the CDA early on were as follows:

- provision of information on dyslexia for the public, teachers, the state bureaucracy and the political leadership;

- education and training of teachers, psychologists and officials;
- provision of diagnostic capability for dyslexia in both the public and private sectors;
- establishment of a policy on dyslexia in the public sector and private schools;
- establishment of a legal framework for state policy;
- establishment of an appropriate state budget for implementation of policy;
- provision of guidance for dyslexics and parents;
- provision of welfare and support services;
- creation of social contact between dyslexic children;
- development of self-esteem by dyslexics;
- provision of remedial education.

The problems of adult dyslexics were acknowledged, but the over-riding priority was considered to be the enlightenment of the population and improvement of education for dyslexic children.

STATE POLICY

The establishment of state policy on dyslexia was considered an urgent problem in view of the almost total lack of knowledge in the state system; this was due to the fact that the Ministry of Education did not have a comprehensive policy on special needs.

One of the key factors in developing a policy on dyslexia was the acceptance by the Ministry of Education of the CDA proposal for a dyslexia committee within the Ministry, with CDA participation. The advantage of this was that the Dyslexia Committee was under the Special Education Service of the Department of Primary Education, which was always much more sensitive to special education problems than the rest of the Ministry. Also because for the first time a committee brought together all the Ministry's departments to examine an issue regarding special education, that of dyslexia. Consequently the departments for primary, secondary and tertiary education participated, as well as the psychology service. A further innovation was the participation of the Ministry of Health in the committee, which allowed the Department of Health psychologist to influence discussion on dyslexia owing to their greater experience in dealing with the problem.

Initially there were disputes as to the terminology to be used, the educational psychologists objecting to 'dyslexia' and agreement being reached on 'special learning difficulties'. Gradually, however, primary education took the lead through officials who had attended conferences on dyslexia and those with special education training, and officials from other departments developed an understanding of dyslexia. A programme for basic training of teachers in dyslexia was introduced on a systematic basis for new teachers at both secondary and primary levels, and the Ministry actively participated in seminars and lectures in towns and settlements throughout Cyprus at the request of the CDA.

THE SPECIAL EDUCATION LAW

The Ministry of Education had been considering since the 1990s a special education law, but despite several reports, no progress had been achieved. Under pressure from the Dyslexia Committee, however, and because of the necessity of adjusting to European

Union norms, the Ministry drafted a Special Education Law, which was given to the CDA and the Federation of Special Needs NGOs for comments in 1998 and was enacted in amended form in 1999.

The enactment of a Special Education Law established the legal basis for dealing with dyslexia in the state education system, and has facilitated the development of private sector policies, but it is obvious that policy goes beyond legal aspects. The law recognizes dyslexia as a disability, establishes a public sector system of diagnosis and committees to determine the classification of a disability as a special need and allows for a liaison officer with schools for the fulfilment of the programme for each child, as determined by experts.

The new law was not brought into operation until the 2001/2002 school year, so it is too early to assess the impact. The situation has been improved but is still far from ideal. Further training on dyslexia and enlightenment of teachers and school directors are required, and guidelines are needed for the education of dyslexic children. The Ministry does not yet have the staff to implement the law properly and there is still confusion as to what measures may be applied to facilitate the examination of dyslexic children. Recently a decision was taken following pressure from the CDA to permit oral examina tions, while the law allows in general for examination conditions such as to permit each child to demonstrate his or her knowledge during examinations.

Unfortunately, however, dyslexia is not considered a special need for the welfare support provided by the Ministry of Labour and Social Insurance. The CDA is now involved in a debate with the Ministry of Labour, with the object of ensuring that low income families obtain support for diagnostic and remedial education, through the normal support proce-dures of the Ministry.

This example demonstrates the difficulties of trying to get inter-governmental co-operation, in order to arrive at a comprehensive policy on dyslexia that incorporates all the state sectors as well as the private sector. It has not yet proved possible to get a policy on dyslexia adopted and implemented across ministries, or to stir up interest in proper monitoring of the private sector. Fortunately most of the private sector is responding quite well to the present rather loose provisions of the Special Education Law, and in some cases the procedures in place are superior to the state sector.

TURKISH CYPRIOT POLICY

Unfortunately the political problems of Cyprus pervade all issues, and the establishment of national policy is almost impossible, given the division of the island, the lack of contact, and the existence from colonial times of a separate Greek Cypriot and Turkish Cypriot education system. Irrespective of the difficulties, the CDA has been able to obtain finan-cial assistance to the sum of $100,000 for the establishment of a Turkish Cypriot Dyslexia Association, and the implementation of common programmes. This was undertaken with the co-operation of the European Dyslexia Association, and has achieved a considerable degree of success under very difficult conditions. On behalf of the CDA, I wish to pub-licly thank Alan Sayles, president of the EDA, for the assistance provided, and University College London for their excellent training programmes. It is planned to assist the Turkish Cypriot association to further the adoption of a comprehensive dyslexia policy, and both associations are now actively seeking ways of further co-operating with the aim of helping the children throughout the island.

CONCLUSION

The main lesson with respect to a policy on dyslexia in Cyprus is that it takes a long time to bring about a change for the better, and it is extremely difficult to establish a comprehensive policy on all aspects of dyslexia. In part, this is because of the difficulties of getting government ministries to listen and act accordingly and, second, to co-ordinate with other ministries. Even co-ordination within ministries is difficult.

In summary, the main conclusions would appear to be as follows:

- Government left to itself will not develop a comprehensive policy on dyslexia.
- Ministries move slowly, require laws and regulations, budgetary approval and tend not to co-ordinate well together.
- The role of the NGO, in this case the Dyslexia Association, is crucial, in part because it is only the NGO that is interested in a comprehensive policy on dyslexia. The role of the NGO should include:
  - enlightenment of the public, officials and politicians;
  - training and information for teachers, welfare and health officials;
  - co-operation with the appropriate ministries;
  - pressure group activity involving officials, state institutions and politicians;
  - co-operation with other NGOs;
  - the role of a general co-ordinator.
- Recognition that dyslexia policy can only be facilitated as a separate category within special needs laws and regulations, and as a special learning difficulty, which results in the need for co-operation with other NGOs to achieve progress.
- Politicians, whether members of parliament or ministers, are concerned about learning difficulties and special needs and can be influenced by NGOs.
- Comments and observations on policy formulation and the drafting of laws have to be well studied and specific, rather than general.
- In promoting policy it is essential to ensure that dyslexia is included, and presented as 'dyslexia' if possible, or otherwise 'special learning difficulty'.
- The media are happy to support enlightenment on dyslexia, because often they get a considerable audience response, which is measurable.
- Active support from the public is essential and this requires enlightenment and education and the provision of support to parents and children.

All these aspects have to be considered together but the key elements appear to be strong public support, enlightenment and education of all concerned, a strong membership base, regular formal and informal contacts with officials and politicians, persistence, patience and determination.

Policy on dyslexia is never completed but requires constant adaptation in order to adjust to research findings, modern demands and experience as to which practices work best.

ORGANIZATION

Cyprus Dyslexia Association
PO Box 23367
Nicosia 1682
Cyprus
Website: dyslexiacy@cytanent.com.cy

CHAPTER AUTHOR

Costas Apostolides
President
Cyprus Dyslexia Association
Email: apostol@cylink.com.cy

DYSLEXIA IN THE CZECH REPUBLIC

Olga Zelinkova

INTRODUCTION

In the Czech Republic about 8 per cent of children are diagnosed with learning disabilities and most of them are children with dyslexia; the number of children with dyscalculia is much lower. About 5 per cent of children suffer from mild learning disabilities.

The Czech Republic uses phonetically highly consistent spelling, making reading in Czech relatively easy. As soon as a Czech child learns the letters of the alphabet and manages to decode and pronounce correctly one letter after another, he or she can correctly read any word at all. If a child does this with sufficient speed, then reading gives the impression of fluency.

From the very beginning, though, the child is taught to combine letters and pronounce whole syllables or words at once. Fluent reading by syllables is also the aim of remedial treatment of dyslexic children. If they attain this level, there is a good chance of their becoming socially acceptable.

The 'socially acceptable' level of reading is a special term which describes fluent reading. It is a rate of approximately 60 to 70 words per minute. Such reading is satisfying for the child, allowing him to enjoy a book and to learn from a textbook by reading efficiently by the end of second grade or at the beginning of the third grade. Comprehension is limited only by the range of the child's vocabulary which, by school age, should be about a thousand words. Reading speed, in these circumstances, is the best individual indicator of reading development. Even accuracy of reading correlates highly with speed.

ASSESSMENT METHODS

The first assessment is usually provided by the school teachers. Teachers observe and monitor the speech and language development, motor development, auditory and phonological levels, and concept of time and space. If it is necessary, they send the child to the Pedagogic Psychological Consulting Centre (PPCC), where there are specialists for learn-

International Book of Dyslexia: A Guide to Practice and Resources. Edited by Ian Smythe, John Everatt and Robin Salter. ISBN 0-471-49646-4. © 2004 John Wiley & Sons, Ltd.

ing disabilities. An assessment at the PPCC should include information about the child's educational, developmental, medical and family backgrounds. After that, the following topics are examined:

- speech and language development, pronunciation, rapid naming, expression, syntax;
- intelligence, motivation, attention and memory;
- perceptuo-motor organization, time and space orientation;
- assessment of oral reading which should include the reading of meaningful text and nonsense sentences. The evaluator analyses fluency, accuracy and speed. Comprehension is assessed using questions or conversation;
- assessment of writing should include copying and writing after dictation. During copying, appropriate pencil grip is observed, use of the right or the left hand, handwriting speed and the form of letters.

Writing from dictation shows not only handwriting but also mastery of language. The analysis of mistakes leads to revealing and detecting their causes. Difficulty with phonemic awareness causes certain omissions or confusions, etc. These mistakes are different from those which are caused by a lack of grammatical awareness. Some children are recommended for neurological or psychiatric assessment or to other specialists.

REMEDIATION/INTERVENTION METHODS: TECHNIQUES AND PROGRAMMES

The therapists or teachers use a multisensory approach together with development. Phoneme–grapheme correspondence is taught and mastered in visual, auditory, and tactile ways and in connection with speech. Several publishers publish books exercise books and teaching aids dealing with the treatment of dyslexia and dyscalculia, for these children. Computer programs for improving reading and writing have recently appeared.

TEACHER TRAINING AND PROFESSIONAL AWARENESS

For teachers in the Czech Republic university education is obligatory. They gain basic knowledge of psychology, sociology, philosophy and, in some specialized fields, also of neurology and neuropsychology. This knowledge then provides a background for the acquisition of new information and problem solving.

Students at the Faculty of Education get basic information about learning disabilities, their diagnosis and treatment. Students of psychology receive training in diagnostics and emotional problems connected with dyslexia. For professionals who are going to work with learning disabled (LD) children, a wide range of courses is available. A variety of lectures are held by members of the Czech Dyslexia Association.

PUBLIC AWARENESS

Czech society is quite well informed about dyslexia and the difficulties connected with it. The first book was published in 1965. Today, articles appear in the professional journals as well as the daily press. Many articles provide new information about this topic. There are also many special programmes on TV and radio.

LEGISLATION, POLICIES AND RESPONSIBILITY

Laws and regulations accepted by the Ministry of Education provide dyslexic individuals with the right to free, appropriate public education, which includes the right to special education and other related services for children with any kind of disabilities. In the public school system there are very few special classes and schools for children with dyslexia. Most dyslexic children are integrated in normal schools.

Special regulations for integrated children refer to the teaching methods, evaluation and assessment. They are taught using other methods appropriate to the individual needs of every child. A child with LD must have an Individual Educational Plan (IEP) which is as similar as possible to the plan of non-disabled children. The child has a support service which is mostly one extra hour of therapy provided by the teacher with special education training or by a teacher who has attended specialized courses.

The IEP is made with the co-operation of the parents, and must identify the annual goals and short-term objectives the student is expected to achieve in one school year. The school's evaluation is more tolerant in comparison to non-disabled children.

THE CZECH DYSLEXIA ASSOCIATION

The Czech Dyslexia Association (CDA) deals with the traditional ideas stated and developed in the 1960s. At that time, the very first classes specializing in dyslexia were adopted and teachers, psychologists and speech therapists started regular meetings in order to exchange their experiences and information about dyslexia. In the 1970s, this group joined the Czech Logopedics Association (Association of Speech Therapists). Seminars were held ten times a year. However, social and economic changes and necessary specialization led to the formation of a separate learning disabilities department.

In 1999 the CDA was registered as an individual organization. Members of the organization are teachers, psychologists, speech therapists, neurologists and even some parents of children with LD or dyslexic adults. The current membership is approximately 300.

The regular seminars usually last all day and are held five times a year. The goal of the seminars is to disseminate new knowledge and experience, and to enable the members to exchange opinions on various problems connected with this topic. In 2001, we managed to start two new projects. One of them is an annual specialized seminar in Brno (the centre of Moravia) which is organized for people living far from Prague. The overall organization is done by people from Moravia (part of the Czech Republic). The second project dealt with the organization as well as the content of the seminar. It took the form of a workshop with the following topics: teaching English to children with dyslexia; course book evaluation; and computer programmes specializing in LD.

The participants of both seminars were very pleased with the results and therefore next year we are going to keep the same structure. A journal of specialized articles has been published by the CDA every year since 1994, and the authors of the articles are members of the association as well as foreign specialists.

The CDA became a member of the European Dyslexia Association in 2001 and the International Dyslexia Association in 2000.

ORGANIZATION

Czech Dyslexia Association
Svatoslavova 17
Prague 4 – Nusle
Czech Republic
Tel: +420 2 691 35 11
Email: zelinkova@mymail.cz

CHAPTER AUTHOR

Olga Zelinkova
Email: zelinkova@mymail.cz

DYSLEXIA IN DENMARK

Birgit Dilling Jandorf, Dorthe Haven and Helen Nielsen

INTRODUCTION

Denmark has a total population of 5.3 million people. The population is said to be relatively homogeneous and this has contributed to consensual approaches to issues including those related to education. Denmark is divided into 13 counties and each county consists of a number of municipalities – 275 in all. There is a rather high degree of autonomy within the counties and the municipalities.

The local authorities have the ultimate responsibility for compulsory school (the *Folkeskole*), including appointments, financial frameworks and curricula. The headteacher has the educational and administrative responsibility for the school, while the teachers have a considerable degree of freedom concerning contents and teaching methods.

THE DANISH EDUCATION SYSTEM

School attendance starts at the age of 7 and there are nine years of compulsory education. A pre-school class is accommodated in the public school and is a preparation for proper school. Children attend pre-school class around the age of 6. Official optional leaving examinations occur after the 9th and 10th Grade. The *Folkeskole* is a unified school in which there is no streaming at any level. Children requiring special consideration are assisted through classroom support and special education.

Secondary education: having attended 9 or 10 years at *Folkeskolen* the pupils may attend three years in upper secondary school (the *Gymnasium*) or in vocational education and training.

Institutions of tertiary education can be divided into universities, university centres, institutions of higher education at university level and other institutions of further education at non-university level.

International Book of Dyslexia: A Guide to Practice and Resources. Edited by Ian Smythe, John Everatt and Robin Salter. ISBN 0-471-49646-4. © 2004 John Wiley & Sons, Ltd.

READING TRADITION AND READING POLITICS

From a historical point of view the attitude towards learning to read has changed. In the 1960s and 1970s the normal opinion was that children were very different regarding how soon they were able to learn to read. It was not very common to distinguish between slow reading development and dyslexia.

In the 1980s and especially in the 1990s, there has been more focus on reading itself. In the international reading survey by the IEA Denmark obtained very low reading rates for the third graders but a little above average for the eighth graders. Consequently it led to an extensive discussion about how to teach children to read in the best way. In the late 1990s the Ministry of Education conducted a national survey that analysed different reading materials in order to find out what method and materials for beginners achieved the best results.

In the last decade much attention has also been paid to 'Early Intervention'. About 98 per cent of all 6-year-old children attend a pre-school class. It is a preparatory class in the same building as the rest of the school. Teaching in a pre-school class was formerly limited to engaging the children in play and other activities promoting the children's development. This vague description is going to be more precisely expressed in connection with statements of objectives for all subjects in the *Folkeskole* including pre-school class, which is about to be implemented by the Minister of Education. The change will emphasize the stimulation of language development in a broad and in a more narrow, phonological sense. Many pre-school teachers already incorporate metalinguistic games and excercises in their teaching with the aim of stimulating pre-school children to discover and attend to the phonological structure of language in order to prepare the children for the reading instruction in first grade.

PREVALENCE OF DYSLEXIA

Dyslexia exists among 3–5 per cent of the population. There has not been a specific survey to confirm this, but according to a national survey 3 per cent of the native population have severe difficulties with common texts such as instructions, documents and narrative texts. No doubt most of these suffer from dyslexia. In the same survey 7 per cent of the participants regarded themselves as dyslexics. The truth may lie somewhere in between. The term 'wordblindness' (*ordblindhed*) is more frequent in Denmark than 'dyslexia', though dyslexia has become more frequent, but most people still tend to say 'wordblindness'.

THE DYSLEXIC PUPIL IN PRIMARY SCHOOL

Special education

The teaching of children, adolescents and adults is regulated by a number of acts, and, with one exception, the general provisions for special education are contained in the ordinary acts applying to the school area in question.

In the *Folkeskole*, where compulsory education is a decisive element of the legislative basis, it is laid down very precisely and compulsorily that all children are obliged and therefore also entitled to complete the *Folkeskole* or other teaching to a standard which can measure up to that of the *Folkeskole*. The Act on the *Folkeskole* thus applies to all children of basic school age as well as children who have not yet started school, if they, due to a handicap, have need of special educational assistance. The aims of the school, the number and scope of the subjects, the organization of the teaching at class levels, evaluation, etc. are thus directed equally at well-functioning pupils and at pupils with severe functional disabilities.

The Act of the *Folkeskole* does, however, contain supplementary provisions on special rights for certain pupils and on possibilities of deviating from some of the provisions in the Act in relation to these pupils. In Section 3 of the Act on the *Folkeskole*, it is laid down that

> Special education and other special educational assistance shall be given to children whose development requires special consideration or upon pedagogical and psychological counselling and upon consultation of the pupil and his/her parents. The provisions on special education and other special educational assistance of the Act on the *Folkeskole* are elaborated on and amplified in a number of ministerial orders and circular letters as well as in a number of guidelines on the content and organization of the teaching. The latter are subject to continuous revision. The regulations governing special education are mainly dealing with the following topics: the pupils, the time of initiating special education and other special educational assistance, the content of the special educational assistance, the different forms of special education, the procedure in relation to referral of pupils to special education and other special educational assistance, special considerations at examinations, transition from school to working life, teacher training, etc. (www.uvm.dk)

COMPENSATION TECHNIQUES

According to the new Act of the *Folkeskole*, new information technology (IT) must be integrated into the teaching of all subjects at all form levels. The knowledge and experience the teachers possess about how to implement IT in their teaching are gradually improving. Concerning dyslexics, the matter has one more point, and it has to do with the grant to obtain the hardware and software.

The school has the responsibility to make necessary special teaching material and IT available for the dyslexic pupil – also if the aids are necessary for homework. It is the school in co-operation with the Pedagogical-Psychological Counselling Service (PPR) and eventually other advisers who evaluate whether a technical aid is necessary or not. The school can also evaluate whether a pupil has to do homework or not, or whether the pupil can do the homework in the school on the computers there.

In some cases an aid is granted as a personal aid according to the Act on Social Services. In that case it is the social worker in the municipality or the local centre for technical aids in the county who is obliged to offer counselling and grant the aid.

The municipal council is responsible for special education and other special educational assistance for children and young people under 18 years of age, who live in the municipality, and whose parents wish them to be enrolled in the *Folkeskole*. The municipal council is furthermore responsible for the provision of special educational assistance to children who have not yet started school.

The county council is responsible for the provision of special education for children and adolescents below 18 years, who live in the county, and whose development calls for special, extensive consideration or support. The county council is also responsible for the provision of special educational assistance to children who have not yet started school.

The municipal council submits a recommendation to the county council about special education and other special educational assistance to children who are enrolled in the schools of the municipality, if the development of the children calls for special extensive consideration or support. It is also the municipal council that recommends that special educational assistance is to be given to children who have not yet started school.

ADMISSION REQUIREMENTS, DIAGNOSIS AND GUIDANCE

There are no objective criteria for establishing the need for special support in the general regulations pertaining to special education, but the procedure for making the decision is described in detail.

As a rule, it is the teacher in the normal school who experiences a given pupil's special needs. It is the Pedagogical Psychological Counselling Service which looks into the nature of the need and makes proposals for remedying it. And it is the headteacher of the school, who decides whether a pupil shall be referred to special education. And finally it is the Pedagogical Psychological Counselling Service that follows the development of the pupil and proposes the necessary adjustments, including the discontinuation of the support.

Special education can be organized in different ways:

- In most cases, the pupil remains in a mainstream school class and receives special education in one or more subjects as a supplement to the general teaching. A pupil may receive special education that replaces the pupil's participation in the normal education in one or more subjects.
- A pupil may alternatively be taught in a special class either within a mainstream school or within a special school.
- And, finally, a combination is possible in which the pupil is a member of either a mainstream school class or a special class, but receives education in both types of classes.

THE DYSLEXIC PUPIL IN SECONDARY SCHOOL AND ADULTS WITH DYSLEXIA

The dyslexic pupil in lower and upper secondary school

Any pupil in Denmark aged 14–18 may attend a lower secondary school, continuation school (*Efterskole*). This is a boarding school of one or two years in the 9th and 10th grade. Approximately 18 of these schools are for dyslexic pupils only. Unlike most of the rest of these schools, the schools for dyslexic pupils do not offer the official leaving examinations, but the pupil may go to their home schools to pass this exam.

After finishing compulsory school, most pupils attend secondary schools. There are a number of different possibilities at this level. Pupils with dyslexia tend to go on to vocational education. Here pupils with dyslexia may receive support for their special needs. The ways in which the support may be given is rather well described by the Ministry of Education. The aid may be either reading tapes, teaching materials on CD-ROM, advanced reading and spelling programmes of synthetic speech.

Nearly one half of the total number of pupils leaving compulsory school continue their education in upper secondary school (the *Gymnasium*). But pupils with dyslexia seem to be more reluctant to follow this educational path. One of the reasons may be that the *Gymnasium* traditionally is considered to be highly academic with lots of reading and writing. Pupils with dyslexia in the *Gymnasium* may receive support of different kinds. Much of the support given is dependent upon the headmaster of the school as there are no explicit rules as to how or how much pupils with dyslexia should be aided.

A special branch of upper secondary school is called the 'Technical Gymnasium'. It is equivalent to the ordinary *Gymnasium* but the subjects are more technically based and that might be the reason why more dyslexic pupils seek this kind of upper secondary education. The possibilities for compensatory aids here are the same as for vocational education in general.

SUPPORT FOR DYSLEXIC STUDENTS IN FURTHER AND HIGHER EDUCATION

Two years ago an Act on special aid for handicapped students enrolled in further and higher education was implemented. For dyslexic students that meant first of all that severe dyslexia now was acknowledged as a handicap along with other handicaps. Second, that students with dyslexia were entitled to receive support in order to put them on an equal footing with students without dyslexia.

SUPPORT FOR PEOPLE WITH DYSLEXIA IN EMPLOYMENT

For people with dyslexia who are employed, the Act on compensation for handicapped people in employment ensures that relevant compensatory aid is provided. It is administered by the handicap consultants employed at the regional public employment services. This Act also includes handicapped people who are self-employed.

ADULTS WITH DYSLEXIA IN GENERAL

The Act on special education for adults ensures that adults with dyslexia may have compensatory special education. Each county is responsible for providing this special education. In each county there is a referral institution and once a dyslexic has been referred to special education, he or she may attend this for free. The compensatory special education may also take place at the local adult education association where a fee has to be paid. The adult need not be referred to this kind of education by other institutions. The compensatory special education for adults is either one-to-one teaching or teaching in small groups – typically 2–4 persons.

Teaching adults with dyslexia may also take place under the Act of preparatory adult education which is teaching in reading skills from level 1 to 4. Special arrangements for dyslexics to join level 1 can be made. This kind of education may also take place at the workplace. The participants are financially compensated when they attend this kind of education.

THE DANISH INFORMATION CENTRE FOR DYSLEXIA

In 1994 the Danish Information Centre for Dyslexia was established together with 11 other information centres for people suffering from different kinds of handicap (stuttering, vision impairment, hearing loss, etc.). The centre is an independent institution funded by the Danish counties. It has a board representing dyslexia research and the Ministry of Education among others. The aims of the centre are to benefit children, adolescents and adults who are at risk of leaving – or who have already left – school with inadequate reading and writing skills. That is done by collecting, processing and communicating current and relevant knowledge about dyslexia.

THE DANISH DYSLEXIA ASSOCIATION (ORDBLINDE/DYSLEKSIFORENINGEN I DANMARK)

The National Dyslexia Association (Ordblinde/dysleksiforeningen i Danmark) was established 60 years ago by the Danish dyslexia pioneer Edith Norrie. Three years earlier she had already established a dyslexia institute, and at that time the relationship between the association and the institute was very close. The Dyslexia Association is one of the oldest in the world and has played an enormous role for many dyslexics and their parents. Its aim is to watch over dyslexics' interests. The association is also represented in the European Dyslexia Association (EDA). In 2000 the association was associated with the Danish Council of Organizations of Disabled People (DSI), which is an umbrella organization.

REFERENCES

Borstrøm, I., Petersen, D.K. and Elbro, C. (1999) *Hvordan kommer børn bedst i gang med at læse?* Copenhagen: Center for Læseforskning, Copenhagen University.
Elbro, C., Møller, S. and Nielsen, E.M. (1991) *Danskernes læsefærdigheder.* Copenhagen: København Undervisningsministeriet og Projekt Læsning, Copenhagen University.
Elley, W.B. (1992) *How in the World do Students Read?* The Hague: The International Association for the Evaluation of Educational Achievement (IEA).

ORGANIZATIONS

The Danish Ministry of Foreign Affairs
Website: www.denmark.dk

The Danish Ministry of Education
Website: www.uvm.dk

Summary of education information on European school systems and policies
Website: www.eurydice.org

The Danish Information Centre for Dyslexia (Dansk Videnscenter for Ordblindhed)
Website: www.dvo.dk

The Danish Dyslexia Association (Ordblinde/dysleksiforeningen i Danmark)
Website: www.ordblind.com

CHAPTER AUTHORS

Birgit Dilling Jandorf (Director), Helen Nielsen (Consultant) and Dorthe Haven (Consultant)
Dansk Videnscenter for Ordblindhed (The Danish Centre for Dyslexia)
Kongevejen 256 A. st.
DK – 2830 Virum, Denmark
Tel.: +45 4595 0950
Fax: +45 4595 0955
Email: dvo@dvo.dk
Website: www.dvo.dk

DYSLEXIA IN EGYPT

Gad Elbeheri

INTRODUCTION

Egypt is one of the oldest civilizations in the world. Seven and a half times the size of Britain, Egypt is situated in the north-east of Africa. With the world's longest river (the River Nile) and one of the world's most important waterways (the Suez Canal), Egypt has both a geographical location and history of which to be proud. Having gained its independence from Britain during the first quarter of the twentieth century, Egypt maximized its efforts to establish a democratic republic. These efforts materialized in 1952, when Egypt was declared an independent Arab state, which is currently known as the Arab Republic of Egypt.

One critical achievement of the government of the newly independent country was to guarantee free education for all Egyptian nationals. The population of Egypt has been increasing ever since and so has the budget of the Egyptian Ministry of Education. With limited resources and ever-increasing ambitions of higher standards of living, most Egyptian nationals view education as a cost-effective means to achieve desirable social change. It is safe to say that this can generally be accomplished through the current generous free educational system that extends to cover university level. Now all individuals in Egypt have access to free mainstream state education, which reflects a strong Arabic influence. There is also a large number of privately run primary and secondary schools across the country in addition to a few private universities. All have a long-standing reputation for delivering a good standard of education that caters for diverse ethnic groups and which focuses on learning foreign languages.

Basic elementary education in Egypt is compulsory and starts at the age of six. Children attend primary schools for five years. Education during this period is conducted in mixed gender classes. After completing the primary stage, children attend preparatory schools. This lasts for three years before finally studying for a further three years in secondary schools should they wish to carry on their education and be considered for a university place. Education in the latter two stages is conducted in single gender classes.

International Book of Dyslexia: A Guide to Practice and Resources. Edited by Ian Smythe, John Everatt and Robin Salter. ISBN 0-471-49646-4. © 2004 John Wiley & Sons, Ltd.

Depending on their secondary school final year marks, students choose from a list of available universities across the country that are commensurate with their personal preferences and their secondary school final marks.

Modern Standard Arabic (MSA) is the official language of the Arab Republic of Egypt as well as being the language of education. A large proportion of Egyptian students, if not all, now have a formative exposure to MSA at school, since school materials and the curriculum are all written in MSA. MSA is also used in modern literary production and in almost all other publications. In addition, MSA is used in the media, both written and broadcast, as well as in formal communications. However similar it might be, Egyptians do not in fact speak Modern Standard Arabic in their everyday situations. They speak Egyptian colloquial Arabic called 'Egyptian national dialect'. Due to the prolific production of Egyptian films, television programmes, and music industries, this qualifies as a second *lingua franca* in the Arab world. To make the situation more complicated, Egyptian colloquial Arabic is also widely used as the medium of instruction within educational settings. In order to appreciate the difference between Modern Standard Arabic, Egyptian colloquial Arabic and other forms of Arabic, let us first examine the nature of the Arabic language.

THE NATURE OF THE ARABIC LANGUAGE

Arabic, the sole or joint official language of some 20 independent countries with an estimated 200 million native Arabic speakers, is a Southern-Central Semitic language. This is a family of genetically related languages that is thought to have developed from a common parent language 'Proto-Semitic', which presumably existed about the 6th/8th millennia BC and was perhaps located in the present-day Sahara. According to Holes (1995), 'The term "Semitic" designates a group of languages, some dead, some still living, and some having a marginal status today as liturgical languages; which all show a sufficient degree of similarity of structure in their phonology and morphology.' Arabic belongs to this Semitic group of languages as spoken in a large area, including North Africa, most of the Arabian Peninsula and other parts of the Middle East. Other living languages of this group are Modern Hebrew, Amharic and other spoken languages of Ethiopia, Aramaic dialects current in parts of Syria and Iraq, and Maltese (Haywood and Nahmad, 1993).

Arabic is an alphabetic language. It is believed to be the second most widely used language in the world, a fact largely due to the Islamic faith (Holes, 1995). The Arabic alphabet is also the second most widely used alphabet in the world, having been adapted to various other diverse orthographies such as Farsi, Urdu, Swahili, Somali, and Ethiopian, to name but few.[1] It is the language of Islam's holy book, the Qur'an (the word itself is a derivative of the Arabic verb 'Qara' to read; hence Qur'an is 'The Reading' or the 'Recitation'), and is therefore the religious and liturgical language of all Muslims, regardless of their origin or mother tongue.

Linguistic literature generally classifies Arabic-speakers as being diaglossic, reserving a 'high' form of the language for formal usage, and using a 'low' form in domestic and casual settings. However, Holes (1995) and Mneimneh (2000) argue that, in effect, more than two separate and distinct forms of the Arabic language are currently in use by each group of speakers, thus a 'polyglossic' (rather than a 'diaglossic') label might be warranted. Holes claims 'the concept of Arabic as a "diaglossic" language, if it was ever accurate, is now a misleading oversimplification (1995, p. 39). Mneimneh (2000) lists four forms, representing main levels, on a vertical continuum:

1 *Classical Arabic* which is used almost exclusively for liturgical purposes, with some further decreasing use in classical literature. Classical Arabic is a highly formalized language that is virtually immune to the pressures of linguistic evolution, and is accepted as the definitive linguistic reference across the Arab world.
2 *Modern Standard Arabic* which derives its syntax, morphology and phonology from Classical Arabic, but is thoroughly infused with terminology and usage inspired and/or adapted from Common European (notably English and French). MSA varies slightly from one Arab locale to another. It is, however, intended as a pan-Arab communication tool.
3 *National dialects* are used in the local media, in the performing arts, and in semi-formal settings. The national dialect of each Arab state is a polished version of its most prestigious sociolect, typically the capital city's elite dialect. While being informed by MSA, the national dialect usually exhibits considerable departure from the Classical Arabic-inspired syntax and phonology. Arabic-speakers are usually capable of understanding the national dialects of adjacent states. Intelligibility, however, decreases with distance.
4 *Local dialects* used in regional and familial settings. Local dialects vary extensively, in all linguistic features, both within each Arab state and across the Arab world. Strung together, they form a horizontal continuum of short-range intelligibility.

ARABIC SCRIPT

The Arabic script evolved probably by the 6th century AD from Nabataean, a dialect of Aramaic current in northern Arabia. It has existed without change since the seventh century AD. Like other Semitic languages, Arabic is written from right to left (Stewart, 1994). The Arabic script is defective: short vowels are not included as independent graphemes in the script but as extra diacritical markings, which are largely neglected, in unvowelled texts. The script is cursive: letters are joined to each other by means of ligatures. The Arabic alphabet is phonemic; it consists of consonants only with the exception of three letters, which are used as long vowels or diphthongs. The Arabic script consists of 17 characters, which, with the addition of dots placed above or below certain characters, provide the 28 letters[2] of the Arabic alphabet.

Arabic, with its 28-letter alphabet, might seem easy enough to learn since it is a phonemic alphabet. Of the 28 named letters of the Arabic conventional alphabet, all but one represent consonantal phonemes (Holes, 1995). But the fact that the script is defective in that short vowels do not appear graphemically in the Arabic script gives rise to different pronunciations of the same phoneme. In order to compensate for this lack of vowels in the script, Arabic makes full use of the diacritical marks. However, these diacritical marks are not used in everyday Arabic, leaving the reader vulnerable to his/her own interpretation and/or understanding of the semantic connotation derived from a given context. According to Holes, this means that 'words with quite different meanings like "darasa" he studied, "durisa" it was studied, "dars" lesson, "darrasa" he taught and "durrisa" it was taught, are homographic in normal handwriting or print' (1995, p. 73). Moreover, letters modify their graphic shape according to their position within the word 'initial, medial, final or isolated from'.

ARABIC MORPHOLOGY

The characteristic feature of Semitic languages is their basis of consonantal roots, which are mostly trilateral. Variations in meaning are obtained by either varying the vowelling of the simple root or by the addition of prefixes, suffixes and infixes. Arabic shows the fullest development of typical Semitic word structure, and therefore should be described with reference to its very complex and productive morphology. Wightwick and Gaafar (1998) argue that the key to understanding how Arabic grammar works is in its system of roots. Once learners understand how roots work, they can start to identify which are the root letters of a word and understand the patterns they produce. They also argue that the learners will then be able to form the different structures following the patterns and use their knowledge to pronounce words correctly and even to guess the meaning of new vocabulary.

THE NATURE OF THE ARABIC LANGUAGE AND DYSLEXIA

From the above brief description of the nature of the Arabic language, one can conclude that Arabic writing is almost entirely phonemic. However,

> the practice of not writing vowels or other orthographic signs with phonological significance (a particular target of educators and script reformers, both Arab and non-Arab) makes it difficult even for educated Arabs to read with complete accuracy unless they have had a thorough grounding in normative MSA. (Holes, 1995, p. 73)

The cursive nature of the Arabic orthography (Arabic characters cannot be handwritten or typed in an independent typeface as their European counterparts), the high number of inflectional morphemes, the irregularity of the Arabic conjugation of verbs and the elaborate use of dots to differentiate between different graphemes (different graphemes assume various shapes depending on their position in the word: initial, medial, final, isolation) are all partially responsible for the manifestations of dyslexia amongst monolingual Arabic speakers. The discrepancy between the Arabic phonology and orthography, though very minimal when compared with another less transparent orthography such as English, notably in the absence of the diacritical marks in the script, is also partially responsible for the manifestations of dyslexia among monolingual Arabic speakers.

LEGISLATION AND POLICIES

Learning disabilities in general, and reading difficulties in particular are a well-documented field of study and research in Egypt (Shehata, 1981; Morsi and Abu Elazayem, 1983; Al Molla, 1987; Othman, 1990; Gilgil, 1995). Local educational authorities in Egypt place great importance on raising awareness of learning difficulties and special educational needs throughout the country. Their efforts have been given a considerable boost due to the hard work of Egypt's First Lady, who personally initiated the 'Reading for all' programme. However, dyslexia is not recognized as a specific reading disability. There is not, as far as we know, a single article in Egyptian law concerning dyslexia. Despite some very few personal initiatives by a handful of academic scholars who recently started research on dyslexia, in general in a country with a population of almost 70 million, dyslexia is hardly a known term. There is no curriculum provision for dyslexia either.

DEFINITION AND TERMINOLOGY

Dyslexia is not recognized as an independent term in either academic or educational circles, nor is it generally defined at the societal level. Special educational needs is being stereotyped in Egypt to include learning handicapped,[3] blind, deaf and hard of hearing individuals, as well as those suffering from aphasia, Down's syndrome, and other severe learning disabilities. No importance is given to dyslexics, simply because the condition is hardly known.

IDENTIFICATION AND ASSESSMENT OF DYSLEXIA

There are currently no methods of identification, assessment or diagnosis for dyslexia available to educational psychologists in Egypt. There are no screening tests for dyslexia available to teachers either. Different methods of assessing and evaluating educational achievements during the academic year and end-of-year exams for students at almost all levels are only *written* as well as being saturated with verbal instructions. Little or no attention is given to oral examinations. Both memorizing by heart and recitation are almost the norms for better achievement.

INTERVENTION AND RESOURCES

Gilgil's (1995) study, as far as we can judge, seems to be one of the first attempts to research dyslexia in Egypt. The research was published in 1995 and fortunately has started to generate some interest among other researchers in Egypt. Now, more researchers are gradually starting to tackle methods of dyslexia assessment, interventions as well as remediation techniques. Although there is a considerable lack of research materials and resources on dyslexia in Arabic, there is a positive move throughout the Arab world to tackle the issue of dyslexia in Arabic. The author is currently working on devising a norm-referenced Arabic dyslexia screening test.

TEACHER TRAINING

So far, there is no formal dyslexia teacher training available in Egypt, although, during professional initial training at university level for student teachers, the topic of learning disabilities is amply discussed. Student teachers at university in Egypt do not come across the issue of dyslexia. Knowledge of 'Learning Difficulties and/or Disabilities' is rather general and is always described in little detail. There are centres for qualified teacher training for teachers of learning-handicapped students. There is a Special Educational Needs Centre at the University of Ain Shams in Cairo.

ADVOCACY GROUPS

There are no specific groups or organizations dedicated to the study or research on dyslexia in Egypt, despite active movements within academic, societal and educational settings regarding special education and learning disability. Hardly a month passes without a conference or a seminar on various aspects of learning disability and special education. There is a newly established non-governmental centre in the heart of Cairo dedicated to the study of learning disabilities in Egypt. The centre is the result of a personal initiative of some Egyptian individuals with a mainly medical background.

EXAM AND CURRICULUM PROVISIONS

The educational system in Egypt depends mostly on the written word, and the Egyptian educational system still regards mis-spelling and poor reading ability as directly related to stupidity and a low level of intelligence. Different methods of assessment during the academic year and end-of-year exams for students at all levels are written as well as being saturated with verbal instructions. There are no exams or curriculum provisions directed at dyslexic individuals in Egypt. Little or no attention is given to oral examinations. Both memorizing by heart and recitation are almost the norms for better achievement, always at the expense of thorough understanding and creative thinking.

ADULT PROVISIONS FOR DYSLEXICS

There are currently no adult provisions for dyslexics available in Egypt.

THE WAY AHEAD

Raising dyslexia awareness through formal education, government policy, advocacy groups and professional organizations is crucial to dyslexic monolingual Arabic speakers. A policy of tolerance towards spelling mistakes due to dyslexia should prevail. Appropriate methods of teaching that address different learning strategies and techniques as well as multi-sensory approaches should be used, particularly with individuals showing signs of dyslexia. The old look-and-say method of teaching should not be the only method available. Awareness of the issue of dyslexia and learning disabilities should be raised. The government of Egypt should adopt new laws and policies to help dyslexic individuals. More government funding is critically needed in the field of dyslexia research.

NOTES

1 The *Encyclopaedia Britannica.*
2 Some linguists consider the Arabic hamza (glottal stop) an independent grapheme that phonologically has a fully functioning consonantal value, which differs from the long vowel alif (first letter of the Arabic alphabet) and therefore the Arabic alphabet should be 29 instead of 28. Others consider the hamza a diacritical mark and hence that it should not be included in the Arabic script.

3 Although one has reservations regarding the use of such a term as being both negative and inappropriate, unfortunately this is the term currently used in Egypt to designate severely learning disabled individuals.

REFERENCES

Al Molla, B.S. (1987) *Delayed Oral Reading, Diagnosis and Remediation*. Riyadh: Aalm Al Kutub Publishing and Distribution.

Gilgil, N. (1995) *Dyslexia: A Diagnostic and Remedial Study*. Cairo: Annahdah Almisriya.

Haywood, J.A. and Nahmad, H.M. (1993) *A New Arabic Grammar of the Written Language*. London: Lund Humphries.

Holes, C. (1995) *Modern Arabic: Structures, Functions and Varieties*. New York: Longman Group Ltd.

Mneimneh, H. (2000) A revolution in the Arab world, linguistic implications of the new information technologies. *Language International*, London: John Benjamins Publishing.

Morsi, M.M. and Abu Elazayem, I. (1983) *Weakness in Reading, Diagnosis and Remediation*. Cairo: Aalm Al Kutub.

Othman, S.A. (1990) *Learning Disabilities*. Cairo: Anglo-Egyptian Publishers.

Shehata, H.S. (1981) Development of oral reading skills in mainstream education in Egypt. Unpublished PhD thesis, Ain Shams University, Cairo.

Stewart, D. (1994) *Arabic Grammar: A Complete Course of Classical Arabic*. London: Darf Publishers.

Wightwick, J. and Gaafar, M. (1998) *Arabic Verbs and Essentials of Grammar*. Chicago: Illinois Passport Books.

CHAPTER AUTHOR

Gad Elbeheri
26 Brookend Rd
Sidcup
Kent DA15 8BE
Email: Gad1318@hotmail.com

DYSLEXIA IN ENGLAND

Carol Orton

THE LEGAL FRAMEWORK

The 1996 Education Act, which applies to England and Wales, sets out specific duties on schools and Local Education Authorities (LEAs) to meet the needs of children who have a learning difficulty. It is a consolidation Act, bringing together all previous and much amended legislation to do with education. In practice, these duties are the same as those first laid out in the 1981 Education Act that followed the Warnock Report of 1978 which investigated the education of handicapped children. Dyslexic adults remember being classified as Educationally Sub-Normal (ESN) or Maladjusted, categories of handicap that existed before the 1981 Act.

The definition of Special Educational Needs (SEN) (see below) swept away the concept of categorizing children with disabilities and learning difficulties. It has sometimes, however, led to a trend against labelling children in any way. Both children and adults identified as dyslexic find the label helps. They often say it is a huge relief to know they are not stupid, something they have invariably thought themselves to be. Moreover, understanding the nature of individual difficulties in learning is often the key to accessing appropriate provision.

Definitions

The 1996 Education Act, Section 312, states that:

> A child has special educational needs if the child has a learning difficulty which calls for special educational provision to be made.
>
> A child has a learning difficulty if:
>
> (a) the child has a significantly greater difficulty in learning than the majority of children of the same age,
>
> (b) the child has a disability which either prevents or hinders use of educational facilities of a kind generally provided for children of the same age in schools within the area of the LEA,

International Book of Dyslexia: A Guide to Practice and Resources. Edited by Ian Smythe, John Everatt and Robin Salter. ISBN 0-471-49646-4. © 2004 John Wiley & Sons, Ltd.

Special educational provision means:
educational provision which is additional to or otherwise different from the educational provision made generally for children of the same age in schools maintained by the LEA (other
than special schools) in the area.

The dyslexic community would argue that dyslexic children have significantly greater
difficulty in learning than their peers and that they require special educational provision.
It has never been that simple. Battle lines are set around how significant a learning difficulty has to be or how large the majority of children of the same age should be. Furthermore, there is a lesser but growing debate about whether dyslexia is a disability.

LEA policies set criteria for deciding when LEA duties step in. More than half the LEAs
surveyed by the British Dyslexia Association (BDA) in 1996 used a model based on a
reading age on or below the 1st percentile. Schools are expected to meet the needs of most
children with special educational needs without any additional support from the LEA.

School governors

School governors have responsibility for all but a small minority of children with SEN.
These responsibilities are, according to Section 317:

(a) to use their best endeavours to secure that if any registered pupil has special educational
needs, the special educational provision that the child's learning difficulty calls for is made,

(b) to secure that the child's needs are made known to all those who teach the child, and

(c) to secure that teachers in the school are aware of the importance of identifying, and providing for, those registered pupils who have special educational needs.

Governors must have regard for the Code of Practice for Special Educational Needs. They
must publish information about their school policy for Special Educational Needs which
must comply with statutory regulations. The policy must describe how the governing body
'evaluates the success of the education which is provided at the school for pupils with
special educational needs' and how resources are allocated 'to and amongst pupils with
special educational needs'.

There has been an abundance of government guidance, reinforced by statutory regulations and changes in legislation since the 1981 Education Act. This would seem to point
to the inability or reluctance of both schools and LEAs to meet special educational needs
effectively.

Statutory assessment

Schools are expected to provide additunal support that matches the needs of their pupils
unless the children have exceptionally severe or complex needs. If the LEA needs to determine the provision for such pupils, they will make a statement of the student's special educational needs. They will do this only after making a formal assessment of the student's
special educational needs. This is not an assessment in the normal 'dyslexia' sense but a
process, lasting up to 18 weeks, involving a gathering of information from agencies that
may be involved with the child.

Either the school or the child's parents can request that the LEA starts an assessment.
If the LEA refuses to assess, the parents can appeal to the Special Educational Needs and
Disciplinary (SENDIS) Tribunal.

The LEA will require evidence on how the school has supported the pupil to date. It is only when a school, having done its best, cannot meet the student's needs that the LEA needs to begin a statutory assessment. There are, inevitably, disagreements between parents, schools and LEAs as to whether it is possible to meet the child's needs.

Statements

Once the LEA has completed the statutory assessment, they must consider 'if it is necessary' to make a statement. If they decide not to do so, parents have a right of appeal to the SENDIS Tribunal.

When LEAs have to determine the provision for children with SEN they make a 'statement' of their needs. The percentage of children with statements varies between LEAs from below 1 per cent to above 5 per cent, with an average of just over 3 per cent.

The statement is a legal document and can ultimately be enforced by the courts. Parents have a right of appeal against the contents of a statement, including the school named on the statement.

The LEA must review the statement at least every 12 months. It may cease to maintain the statement but should only do so after consultations with the parents, who have a right to appeal to the SENDIS Tribunal.

THE SEN TRIBUNAL

The SENDIS Tribunal is independent and made up of a lawyer chair and two wing members with expertise in SEN. Its decisions are binding on both parents and LEAs. It hears nearly 2,000 cases a year, about a third on 'literacy difficulties including specific learning difficulties'. Over 60 per cent of appeals are won, at least in part, by parents.

Parents

It will be clear from the above that parents have considerable rights once statutory processes start. However, these only happen for a tiny minority of children. Within schools the Code of Practice for SEN stresses the value of information from parents and the child, and strongly encourages a working partnership between school and home. LEAs have to provide a Parent Partnership Service. New in 2002 is a requirement for LEAs to have a Disagreement Resolution Service to avoid or resolve disputes between parents and LEAs or schools about their child's special educational provision. This service must include an independent element using mediators not employed by the LEA.

DYSLEXIA-FRIENDLY SCHOOLS

Just after the first Code of Practice for SEN was published, in 1994, the British Dyslexia Association (BDA) organized a series of conferences for Special Educational Needs Co-ordinators (SENCOs) and school governors. Neil Mackay, SENCO at Hawarden High School in North Wales, explained how, by developing a 'dyslexia-friendly school' and implementing whole school policies, children's needs could be met. Realizing that he could not provide individually for the dyslexic pupils in the schools he turned his efforts to training subject teachers. As SENCO, he then had time to provide specialist teaching for those still needing it.

In 1997 the City and County of Swansea (Wales) faced both a deficit in its SEN budget, and angry parents and frustrated teachers. They embarked on an authority-wide 'dyslexia-friendly' policy. This involved training a specialist teacher for every school by 2002. The policy won the confidence of parents and the enthusiasm of schools. The management of SEN finance was applauded by the District Auditor.

In England the notion of a 'dyslexia-friendly school' exists in small pockets of good practice, usually where a charismatic specialist teacher holds a position of some authority within a school. Two English LEAs, East Sussex and Staffordshire, are committed to the ethos of dyslexia-friendly schools and setting up training for specialist teachers.

The relationship between schools and LEAs in England is subtly different to that in Wales, where recent legislation has not been implemented fully because powers passed to the Welsh Assembly have not been used. In England, schools can operate much more individually unless they are failing. Funding for training, including training for the SEN, is delegated to schools on a much larger scale which means that if a school has other priorities then SEN and dyslexia can be met with token provision. The situation is not helped by the publication of league tables of schools' results. Nevertheless, where there is the will and the skill within their school, dyslexic children can thrive.

The BDA published its *Achieving a Dyslexia Friendly School* resource pack in 1999, funded by the Department for Education and Employment (now Department of Education and Skills). Over 50,000 copies have so far found their way into schools and is now in its third edition. One of the BDA's current objectives is that 25 per cent of all schools will be working towards dyslexia-friendly status by 2004.

THE DISABILITY DISCRIMINATION ACT

The SEN and Disability Act 2001 brought education within the Disability Discrimination Act (DDA) 1995. At the time education was explicitly excluded. The definition of disability differs considerably from that of SEN, i.e. 'A person has a disability if he has a physical or mental impairment which has a *substantial* and long-term *adverse* effect on his ability to carry out *normal day to day* activities.' Schools and colleges cannot discriminate against a person with a disability for a reason to do with their disability and must make reasonable adjustments to try and accommodate them, both for admissions and the education on offer. The SEN Tribunal was expanded to become the SEN and Disability Tribunal to hear cases relating to disability discrimination.

The associated Code of Practice for schools and another for further and higher education gave examples of situations that may be regarded as discriminatory. Some of these refer specifically to dyslexic children and students. Others address situations commonly experienced by dyslexic children and students, for example entrance examinations. Since the Codes accept dyslexia as a disability and promote the reasonable adjustments necessary to avoid discrimination some of the things that repeatedly happen with dyslexic children (being put in low sets, punished for failing to copy off the board, etc.) may finally become a thing of the past. The 'dyslexia-friendly school' has already eliminated them.

Where parents feel discrimination has taken place, they will be able to appeal to the SEN Tribunal, now renamed the SENDIS Tribunal. This will not have to wait for an LEA decision, as for appeals associated with the 'statementing' process. The Tribunal will be able, for disability appeals, to make 'any decision it sees fit' including ordering an apology or a change in school policy. Students take their complaints through the courts and may ask for financial compensation.

The Act requires LEAs to have an Accessibility Strategy and schools to have Accessibility Plans that spell out their plans to increase access to

- Increasing the extent to which disabled pupils can participate in the curriculum
- Improving the physical environment to increase the extent to which disabled pupils can take advantage of education and associated services and
- Improving the delivery of information to disabled pupils which is provided to pupils who are not disabled – taking into account views of pupils and parents

FURTHER AND HIGHER EDUCATION

It is somehow more acceptable to be dyslexic when a child becomes a student in further or higher education. Prospectuses advertise the skills of their Learning Support Departments, though good practice is not by any means universal. The law is much less prescribed though colleges lose funding if students drop out.

For dyslexic adults seeking to improve their basic skills, the outlook is more gloomy. There is a considerable push to attract adults to literacy and numeracy classes but the agencies providing the courses have not yet accepted that a high proportion of their students may be dyslexic. Dyslexic adults who have tried have reported the humiliation of failing yet again. On the other hand, some have discovered their dyslexia at a Basic Skills class and been passed onto specialist advice and support.

TOWARDS SOCIAL INCLUSION

While the law looks at individual difficulties and individual provision, the prevailing view of those individuals is that the institutions themselves need to change. The 'dyslexia-friendly school' is a massive step in this direction.

Although practice is slow to change, one hopeful sign is the way in which the phrase 'dyslexia friendly' has become part of everyday jargon among a growing number of organizations. The challenge is to make the language real.

USER GROUPS IN ENGLAND

The British Dyslexia Association was established in 1972 by a group of local associations, and has become the main organization for parents and teachers of dyslexic children. As an advocacy organization, it has both supported the individual and attempted to influence policy at the government level. It is an umbrella organization, controlled by its council members, which includes local groups and corporate members, including dyslexia teaching centres. As it is a representative user organization, most other English groups and organizations can be found on the BDA website. It has a comprehensive range of publications, including the tri-annual *Dyslexia Contact* magazine, and the annual *Dyslexia Handbook*.

There are also a number of independent groups concerned with the adult dyslexic, the largest of which is the Adult Dyslexia Organisation.

ORGANIZATIONS

British Dyslexia Association
98 London Road
Reading
RG1 5AU
Tel.: 0118 966 2677
Email: admin@bda-dyslexia.demon.co.uk
Website: www.bda-dyslexia.org.uk

Adult Dyslexia Organisation
336 Brixton Road
London SW9 7AA
Tel.: 020 7737 7646
Email: dyslexia.hq@dial.pipex.com
Website: www.futurenet.co.uk/charity/ado/

Dyslexia Institute
Park House
Wick Road
Egham
Surrey
TW20 OHH
Tel.: 01784 222300
Email: hqreception@dyslexia-inst.org.uk

CHAPTER AUTHOR

Carol Orton
Recently Policy and Local Services Director,
British Dyslexia Association.
Email: Carol.Orton@redbridge.gov.uk

DYSLEXIA IN FINLAND

Heikki Lyytinen, Mikko Aro and Leena Holopainen

INTRODUCTION

In Finnish, reading and writing difficulties are usually referred to using a common abbreviation *lukihäiriö*, i.e. reading and writing disorder. This underlines the finding that reading and spelling problems usually seem to go hand in hand. Most children with this disorder end up being quite accurate although slow in reading but usually are still prone to minor spelling errors. These are often seen in the context of short and long phonemes spelled with one and two subsequent same graphemes, respectively (e.g. *mato* vs. *matto*, *tuli* vs. *tuuli*).

THE POSITION OF INDIVIDUALS WITH DYSLEXIA IN FINLAND

There is no official definition or special legislation relating to dyslexia, but about 10 per cent of children who are slow in learning to read receive special attention in school from specially trained teachers. Pupils whose educational problems are considered to be relatively mild (e.g. reading, writing or speech disorders) may receive this help in the form of part-time special education within the course of normal instruction. Little support is available following basic education, although there are a few trained teachers in some vocational schools who are able to help individuals with dyslexia. The awareness of those secondary school teachers who are not specialized in special needs is low. Dyslexia can create great difficulties for the individual in the later stages of education. This is because the receipt of support for dyslexic problems is highly dependent on the activity of the individual and on the resources that happen to be available. In the matriculation exam, which is a national test after high school and an important factor for university admission, dyslexia is only taken into account if specifically asked for beforehand. However, this

International Book of Dyslexia: A Guide to Practice and Resources. Edited by Ian Smythe, John Everatt and Robin Salter. ISBN 0-471-49646-4. © 2004 John Wiley & Sons, Ltd.

status has only a cosmetic effect on the marking of the exam. There is some training available in adult evening schools but too little to fulfil the required needs.

Although reading and writing problems are common in primary schools, they have received relatively little public attention. Minimal support is available for adults with dyslexia. In recent years the emergence of societies for individuals with learning disorders (Erilaiset oppijat-yhdistys, Association of Different Learners) has helped in the raising of public awareness. Similarly, the increase in research activity (e.g. in the Niilo Mäki Institute, University of Jyväskylä) has made it possible to initiate networking between people working in the area, researchers and individuals who have problems related to literacy.

REMEDIATION IN SPECIAL EDUCATION

In primary and secondary schools, children with reading and writing disabilities receive help in the form of part-time special education administered by special teachers. In the case of severe learning problems, the child can obtain special help before school age from a number of sources. These include kindergarten teachers specially trained in early support, psychologists, speech therapists or physicians in central hospitals, local health care centres, family guidance centres or in the learning disability support centres (such as the Niilo Mäki Institute in Jyväskylä). These services are also available at school age although they vary according to the location of the school. Some of these services are available only in large towns. However, unless the pupil has additional problems in spoken language skills, it is relatively rare for the remediation of problems associated with dyslexia to be available outside the school setting.

The remediation of reading and writing disabilities in schools is based on the structure of the language, and the role of syllables is important. At the basic level, special education begins with the teaching of letter–sound correspondences and continues step by step towards phonemic segmentation and the assembly of CV and VC syllables. It then proceeds gradually towards more complex syllabic structures and syllabic assembly. Reading and writing skills are taught simultaneously. Special teachers use multi-sensory methods, key-word pictures and stories to teach the names and sounds of the letters. Analogies (drill-method) are used for the mastery of each syllable structure, e.g. MAA-SAA-LAA. Special attention is paid to the syllabification of words that include long phonemic quantities, as in these words the phonemic output is not always accurate. When mastery of syllable structure has reached the level which allows fluent word decoding, more attention is paid to reading comprehension and reading strategies.

ASSESSMENT OF READING AND WRITING DISABILITIES IN SCHOOLS

In Finnish schools, special education for dyslexia is based on the individual assessment of pupils' achievements, abilities and disabilities. Assessment is usually made jointly by the primary school teacher and the special teacher. Three different methods are used to assess pupils' reading and writing abilities at school. The first and most common is 'indicative' and is based on the pupil's reading and writing output. In this kind of assessment, the pupil's production indicates the problems in their reading and writing. The usual indications are the quality of reading and writing errors, and reading speed. The second way of assessing a pupil's abilities is based on reading and writing processes. There are numerous cognitive models of reading and writing which delineate the relevant processes and a common feature of many is that reading and writing are divisible into sub-processes. The special teacher assesses the mastery of these processes. The third part of the assessment concentrates on attempts to uncover the background of the disorders. This final part of the assessment is usually carried out in co-operation with a psychologist. Because there are no official criteria for admission into special education, the assessment procedures have been quite varied. During the 1990s, many new tools for the assessment of reading and writing development emerged, for example, in decoding, reading comprehension, phonological awareness, and handwriting. The first stringent standardized reading test was published in 1998 and includes group tests, which measure phonological skills, decoding and reading comprehension. Relatively little research relating to the assessment of Finnish reading skills has been published. Only a recent development in university research units has initiated research, which relates to extensive validation and standardization of reading tests in the areas of both decoding and comprehension.

TEACHER TRAINING

Special education for children with reading and writing disabilities has taken place in Finnish primary schools since 1967, when the first special teachers graduated. Primary school teachers, who embark on the one-year special teacher training (organized in three universities in Finland), must already have completed basic studies in special education in addition to their MA degree. The basic studies include literacy, lectures, and practical demonstrations encompassing different areas of special education. When attending special teacher training, the student can choose the field of special education with which they particularly want to become acquainted (e.g. reading, writing and language disabilities, social-emotional problems or general learning disabilities).

An alternative to special teacher training is also available. Students can graduate directly with the MA degree in special education without a primary school teacher qualification. This course lasts for four years and includes studies in general special education in the first two years, and, as with the aforementioned special teacher training, the student can choose a speciality field of special education in the final two years of the course. These two types of special teachers work in primary and secondary schools.

In upper secondary schools, the provision of special education services has been minimal. Recently, some courses have been organized for mother-language teachers in vocational schools to enable them to help pupils with learning disabilities. These one-year courses have been organized to train personnel for this purpose by the Department of Special Education at the University of Jyväskylä and the Vocational Teacher Training College's Continuing Education Centres. The legislative goal has been that every young adult with dyslexia should be able to benefit from individual guidance in their vocational studies. The Continuing Education Centres in most Finnish universities organize relatively extensive (about three years on a part-time basis) continuing special education for primary school and special teachers in those fields of special education in which they may want to expand their knowledge.

ORGANIZATION

HERO
Wilhelmsgatan 4 B 13
00100 Helsingfors
Finland
Tel.: +358 9 6869 3500

CHAPTER AUTHORS

Heikki Lyytinen and Mikko Aro
Department of Psychology
University of Jyväskylä
Finland
Leena Holopainen
Niilo Mäki Institute
Finland
Email: Heikki.Lyytinen@psyka.jyu.fi

DYSLEXIA IN FRANCE

Myriam Risser

INTRODUCTION

Until very recently, the existence of 'dyslexia' was not officially acknowledged in French schools. Nevertheless, individual initiatives have existed in places for some years, but only a few dyslexic children had the benefit of these local initiatives.

THE SCHOOL SYSTEM IN FRANCE

In French primary schools, there is a team of class teachers, each one having the responsibility to teach a class. Classroom assistants, Special Educational Needs (SEN) teachers, SEN coordinators and a SEN budget do not exist. If a class teacher feels unable to deal with the difficulties of a pupil, he or she can request help from the RASEDs.[1] These are support services located in one of the largest schools in the district. Three types of professionals work there: educational psychologists, special teachers and educators. They may intervene in the school where they are needed. The dyslexic child is then withdrawn from his class to work with one of these professionals for half an hour or an hour per week in a one-to-one session or in small groups with other under-achieving children. Otherwise, the child goes for half a day or a day per week to an 'open class' located in the school where the RASED has its headquarters.

Two main problems appear at this level:

- There are not enough special services and they do not have enough professionals: three professionals for as many as 500 or 700 pupils. Some schools are not part of a RASED.
- Nobody has special training to support dyslexic children. Some educational psychologists even deny the existence of dyslexia.

The RASED does not operate at the secondary education level, but during their first year in secondary schools, subject teachers provide support hours to pupils having difficulties in French and/or maths.

International Book of Dyslexia: A Guide to Practice and Resources. Edited by Ian Smythe, John Everatt and Robin Salter. ISBN 0-471-49646-4. © 2004 John Wiley & Sons, Ltd.

Within some schools, special classes[2] have been created, but they are designed for those suffering from mental or motor handicaps, visual or hearing impairments and not for dyslexic children.

TEACHER TRAINING

During their initial training, the class teachers (at primary or secondary education levels) do not receive any formal training in dyslexia. With respect to in-service training, they may have the opportunity to hear a lecture about the subject organized by an association, the school or the Regional Education Authority, but it is not possible to become a specific learning difficulties/dyslexia teacher. These courses do not exist in France, even for those working in the RASEDs.

IDENTIFICATION, ASSESSMENT AND SUPPORT

In 1999, a team of researchers[3] from the Regional Education Authority of Grenoble published an evaluation that aims to screen out the children at the end of the nursery school (5–6 years old), who have not acquired the necessary skills to learn reading and writing in primary schools. Input from the class teachers and the parents is required to obtain constructive measurements. However, the use of these tests is not compulsory. Educational psychologists from the RASED can be requested by the class teacher to assess a pupil, but formal tests are not used in the identification of dyslexia.

In fact, if the parents or the teachers suspect that a child has a learning difficulty, a speech therapist has to be consulted for assessment and adequate support for approximately half an hour or an hour per week. Speech therapists are mostly independent workers and they do not intervene in the schools. Half of the cost of their consultations is paid for by the Social Security and mutual health insurances, but parents will have to transport their children there.

In a CMPP,[4] a team of psychologists, special teachers, educators, speech therapists and doctors can also provide assessment and support; however, they intervene rather on a psychological basis. These centres are run by the Health Minister and their services are free of charge but there is only one in each large town.

THE WAY AHEAD

In 2000, the Education Ministry asked for a report on the situation of dyslexic children in French schools. Following the findings, an Action Plan was issued in March 2001. It prescribed 28 measures to put in place between June 2001 and December 2003. The actions involve both the Educational and Health Ministers. The measures are based on five fields of priorities: prevention, identification, provision, professional awareness and the application of the Plan itself.

For instance, before the end of 2001, class teachers and school doctors should have the adequate tools to evaluate the children during their last year in nursery school and their first year in primary school (6–7-year-old children), while school doctors from the health services would screen children as soon as they enter nursery school at the age of 3–4 years. The national tests already applied at the entry of the third year of primary school and the first year of secondary school should be modified in order to highlight specific learning difficulties. However, most of these tools and tests have still to be developed.

Regarding provision, speech therapists will remain the main interveners, but, at both primary and secondary education levels, special classes for dyslexic children will be formed but the pupils will attend them only for a few hours per week, according to their needs. Special units should be created in some hospitals to support children suffering from severe dyslexia. In addition, Regional Councils will have officially to determine who is competent to support dyslexic children and under what conditions. Special provisions for examinations will be established: no details are given but even now it is difficult to obtain extra time for a dyslexic child.

One of the greatest tasks will be to develop professional awareness of all those involved in the educational fields as well as doctors, speech therapists, social workers and other health service professionals. But first of all, skilled instructors must be trained in order to teach all those concerned in the education of dyslexic children.

To summarize, the Action Plan aims to make up for the delay the country has experienced regarding dyslexia matters. Certainly, it is a great achievement to define the issues and the Action Plan seems to put effective measures in place. However, it is not law and the impact of a change in government cannot be foretold.

France has just started on a long road towards discovering dyslexia and all those concerned know that many years are needed to ensure a happy and successful schooling of our dyslexic children. On the other hand, nothing has been planned for students in higher education or for adults. They can go to a speech therapist as the youngest do and try on their own to do their best in life.

APEDA FRANCE

APEDA (Association de Parents d'Enfants en Difficulté d'Apprentissage du langage écrit et oral: Association of Parents having a Child with Specific Learning Difficulties) France was created in 1982 by parents of dyslexic children. For years, it campaigned to obtain the recognition of dyslexia as a learning difficulty by the educational system. The Action Plan represents a long-awaited achievement, but one has to remain cautious and active to ensure its application throughout the country as well as its continuity through the years. APEDA France participated in the foundation of the UNFD (Union Nationale France Dyslexie: French National Union of Dyslexia) in 1986 and in 1997 became a member of the FLA (Fédération Française des Troubles Spécifiques du Langage et des Apprentissages: French Federation of Language and Specific Learning Difficulties), which brings together parents and professional associations. Through its lobbying, it has played an important part in the recent events. In 1987, APEDA France was also one of the associations that participated in the foundation of the European Dyslexia Association.

NOTES

1 Réseau d'Aide Scolaire d'Education Spéciale: Network of Educational Support and Special Education.

2 These are integration classes called CLIS at the primary level and UPI at the secondary level.
3 Research conducted by Michel Zorman.
4 CMPP: Centre Médico Psychopédagogique: Medical, Psychological and Educational Centre.

ORGANIZATIONS

APEDA France
3 bis, Avenue des Solitaires
78320 Le Mesnil St Denis
France
Website: www.ifrance.com/apeda/

FLA
43, Avenue de Saxe
75007 Paris
France
Email: federation.fla@aol.com

Coridys
7 Av. Marcel Pagnol
F-13090 Aix-en-Provence
France
Tel.: +33 4 4295 1796
Email: coridys@club-internet.fr
Website: www.coridys.asso.fr/

Union Nationale France Dyslexie et Dysphasie
28 Av. Arnold Netter
F-75012 Paris
France
Tel.: +33 173 6410 or +33 173 6061

CHAPTER AUTHOR

Myriam Risser
9 rue des Champs
68130 Carspach
France
Email: r.myriam@wanadoo.fr

DYSLEXIA IN GERMANY

Christiane Löwe and Gerd Schulte-Körne

INFLUENCE OF THE *LÄNDER*

The Bundesrepublik Deutschland consists of 15 *Länder* and the capital Berlin. The historical development of Germany out of many small kingdoms and dukedoms into a nation left some of the former sovereignty to the *Länder*, some of it went to the Bundesrepublik. Within the context of this chapter the complete sovereignty of each *Land* (plural: *Länder*) in all educational and cultural aspects (*Kulturhoheit*) is the most important one. As each *Land* can decide on its own educational system, the Bundesrepublik shows a variety of educational possibilities, all of which have their advantages as well as their disadvantages. The 15 Ministers of Education meet regularly in the Kultusministerkonferenz (conference of Ministers of Culture and Education). One of their aims is to find a certain amount of conformity within the German system, but at the same time try to maintain the individual characteristics of each *Land*. Of course, different aspects of the pedagogical approach to the education of dyslexic children find their supporters within the different educational ministries. Therefore the variety of the help given to dyslexic children within the school system is enormous. All *Länder* have drawn up and issued regulations on the support children with reading and spelling difficulties should get. In some *Länder* there are regular special needs lessons within normal teaching hours, in other *Länder* there is no support from school at all. In these *Länder* the support the children need is solely given outside school.

REMEDIATION

Beyond these aspects there are various and far-reaching tendencies to give the Bundesrepublik a set framework of guidelines for the education of dyslexic children. The Kultusministerkonferenz is in the process of drafting new general rules for the help dyslexic children should find within their school system. For obvious reasons these guidelines will

International Book of Dyslexia: A Guide to Practice and Resources. Edited by Ian Smythe, John Everatt and Robin Salter. ISBN 0-471-49646-4. © 2004 John Wiley & Sons, Ltd.

have to be on a very general level as they must not interfere with each *Land's* individual system. The possibilities which teachers offer today vary widely from additional work for the children to take home to special needs tuition within the classroom for a few minutes every day. There are two mainstream methods for remediation for dyslexic children in Germany which have been shown to be effective: training phonological awareness and rule-based spelling training. However, methods which have not yet been evaluated, such as training of basic visual and auditory perception, are very common, mainly in tuition outside school.

School tutoring takes place during German lessons in the classroom or in groups of five to six children outside normal school hours. Unfortunately, these groups are not as homogeneous as they should be to influence the effect of learning to read and spell. Children with reading and spelling problems due to problems arising from being bilingual and children with attention deficit syndrome are treated together with dyslexic children, although for each group specialized interventions are recommended.

The kind of help a teacher offers or can offer obviously depends greatly on their professional training. The knowledge of special needs tuition is still not part of the areas of learning which teachers training colleges require for their final exams. Even though the demand by the general public on the school and the teachers has been growing enormously within the past ten years, the diagnosis of dyslexia within the first two school years remains difficult. High diagnostic uncertainty frequently arises because of different intra-individual reading and spelling development. Furthermore, teachers are absolutely free to decide which methods to use for their reading and spelling teaching. Depending on the method they choose, there is a high inter-class individuality in reading and spelling development. Thus for a reading and spelling disorder, a valid diagnosis can be attempted from the end of the second grade. In Germany depending on the legislation of the *Länder*, diagnosis is performed by a specially trained physician (child and adolescent psychiatrist) or a school psychologist or teacher. Diagnostic procedures vary greatly depending on whether a teacher or a medically trained professional is responsible for the tests performed.

PRIVATE TUITION

A major problem for parents arises after dyslexia has been diagnosed: how do they find appropriate help for our child? As mentioned above, there are a few *Länder* where the school system is such that help within the school and daily school life can be offered successfully. But in most *Länder* the parents will have to find help outside the school. A vast field of private tuition has opened up in the last years. Many of these institutions offer help on a high and qualified level, but unfortunately this does not hold true for all of them.

DYSLEXIA IN ADULTS

In contrast to the high public awareness of dyslexia in German children, the existence of dyslexia in adults has been ignored. Recent investigations of university students have found that about 2–5 per cent of the students are reported to have spelling and reading problems. However, many dyslexic adults still are not identified. Specialized aid, e.g. for dyslexic students or employees, is not available.

ADDITIONAL SOURCES OF INFORMATION

Research is encouraged and political decisions are supported by the German Dyslexia Association (Bundesverband Legasthenie – GDA). In this association parents, teachers, academics and all people concerned with the topic try to improve all ranges of dyslexia, beginning with early symptoms during nursery years, continuing through school life and helping during the early professional years of a dyslexic. Support is provided through the 16 local Dyslexia Associations (*Landesverbände*) affiliated to the GDA. The *Landesverbände* are independent registered charities. They hold meetings with or without invited guest speakers, run courses, and offer literature for sale and to borrow. One of the major tasks of the local working groups is to provide access to the local facilities for assessment and tuition. Additionally, they frequently provide a local telephone help-line.

There is a large and continuously growing range of literature to help in everyday problem situations available to the general public from the Bundesverband. GDA members receive local and national dyslexia information including the GDA magazine *Legasthenie* four times a year. Furthermore, the Bundesverband organizes at regular intervals one of Europe's biggest conferences on dyslexia. The conference brings together highly qualified scientists and the general public, a forum which will allow contacts normally not possible.

ORGANIZATION

Bundesverband Legasthenie e.V.
Königstrasse 32
30175 Hannover
Germany
Tel: +49 511 31 87 38
Email: info@legasthenie.net
Website: www.legasthenie.net

CHAPTER AUTHORS

Christiane Löwe
Gerd Schulte-Körne
Dyslexia Research Group
Department of Child and Adolescent Psychiatry and Psychotherapy
Philipps-University Marburg
Hans-Sachs-Strasse 6
35039 Marburg
Germany
Email: Schulte1@med.uni_marburg.de

DYSLEXIA IN GREECE

Maria Sp. Mazi, Styliani Nenopoulou and John Everatt

THE GREEK WRITING SYSTEM

Although Greek has a more transparent orthography than some writing systems, such as English, it is not entirely regular in its correspondence between phoneme and grapheme. For example, different letters are sometimes used to represent the same sound; h, i and u all represent an 'ee' sound (as in 'feet') within different words. Also, combinations of letters are used to represent the same sounds; e.g., that 'ee' sound is also represented by 'ei' or 'oi' within different words, while the simpler 'e' (as in 'pen') sound can be represented by 'ai' as well as 'e'. The reverse situation, where the same letter can represent different sounds, can also be found. Hence 't' can be sounded as 't' in some instances and 'd' in others. If 't' follows 'n' in the middle of a word, a simple rule is to sound it out as 'nd' (*entaxei*), but not in 'exception' words such as *antio*, where it should be sounded as 'd'. And there are, of course, the bane of all poor spellers, examples of letters within words which remain more or less silent (e.g., the letter 'u' in *euboia*). Thus, although Greek may not be as obscure in its spelling–sound correspondences as some written forms, such as English or French, it is by no means an entirely shallow orthography.

PROBLEMS IN LEARNING TO READ/WRITE GREEK

Porpodas (1989; 1990) explains that such inconsistencies in the Greek spelling system were the result of a historical change (from old to modern Greek) that occurred in the pronunciation of some phonemes, which has not led to a corresponding change in the letter symbols. The consequence of these changes is that learners of the Greek writing system will probably find reading easier than spelling. Given such complexities in the Greek written form, it is not surprising to find some children experiencing great difficulty in acquiring literacy. Indeed, the official Greek *Information Manual of Special Education*

International Book of Dyslexia: A Guide to Practice and Resources. Edited by Ian Smythe, John Everatt and Robin Salter. ISBN 0-471-49646-4. © 2004 John Wiley & Sons, Ltd.

(1994) suggests that 5 per cent of children in Greece are dyslexic. However, many researchers and practitioners bemoan the dearth of reliable statistical data on the incidence of dyslexia (and dysgraphia, since it is often argued that Greek is much harder to write than read) within the Greek population.

LEGISLATION AND PROVISIONS

The special education sector is considered relatively new in the Greek educational system, although the respective legislation was initially introduced as early as 1972. A brief overview of legislation can be found in the Greek Ministry of Education and Religious Affairs (1994). It is only during the past 20 years that significant steps have been taken for the organization and operation of special education within the Greek educational system. The official Greek *Information Manual of Special Education* (1994) indicates that there are two basic forms of provision for individuals with learning difficulties (which includes those with dyslexia, language problems, etc.). The first includes special classes within mainstream schools up to the age of 13; the second, special schools or institutions, which often involve more prolonged remediation and boarding. Children with learning difficulties usually attend special classes for only a few hours per week; the remainder of their schooling is spent in mainstream primary school classes. There is no doubt that the number of such special classes has dramatically increased in the past two decades. In the late 1970s, there was no official record of them. Most children with learning difficulties had to manage as best they could within mainstream schools. By the mid-1990s, there were over 600 special classes; the dramatic increases being in the late 1980s/early 1990s as awareness of the problem increased. However, whether a child is offered help within a special class may depend upon geographical location, rather than the child's needs. The vast proportion of special classes are situated in large cities (e.g., Athens may possess as many as 30 per cent), with many smaller cities and islands reporting none. Even if such a special class does exist within their school or immediate vicinity, a dyslexic child may not profit if the remedial teacher lacks training and if large class sizes result in limited time being available for working with the remedial teacher. Although there are a number of courses for teachers, they frequently complain of a dearth of training and official guidance.

The recent Act (2817/2000) for Special Education introduced some new important elements in the overall structure of the system:

1 Establishment of Centres of Diagnosis, Assessment and Support (CDAS), based in the capital city of each prefecture, with main responsibilities for the recording of any problems of special education within their catchment areas, the organization and administration of the enrolment procedures in the special education schools of the prefecture, the continuous monitoring of standards in these schools, the provision of full support and guidance for the teaching staff and parents alike, and the publication of proposals for the improvement of the system (teaching methods, assessment procedures, technical infrastructure, etc.). For the smooth operation of these Centres new specialist teachers will be recruited, from a wide variety of disciplines (sociologists, social workers, psychologists, paedo-psychiatrists, speech therapists, deaf-education specialists, administrative personnel, etc.). (Art. 2, par. 3–10)

2 Establishment of a new Department of Special Education within the Greek Pedagogical Institute.

3 Introduction of strict new demands for the recruitment of teachers in special schools (post-graduate studies, special training certificates, long experience in related fields, etc.). (Art. 4, par. 1)

4 Establishment of Regional Directorates of Education, which will assume overall responsibility for any organizational aspect of public and private schools within each region (Art. 14, par. 29), something that so far had been the responsibility of the prefectural authorities. In that sense, a 'centralization' of the whole system – not only of that of special education – and the stripping of powers of the (elected) prefectural authorities in favour of the regional branches of the central government are under way.

DIAGNOSIS AND REMEDIATION

The development and assessment of remediation practices is an area in need of further work. Diagnosis of learning difficulties can be made in many public Greek hospitals as well as by private practitioners and/or educational psychologists in private dyslexia centres or institutions, with some also providing treatment regimes (see also Organizations below). The University of Patras operates a centre for the diagnosis and treatment of dyslexia headed by Professor Constantine Porpodas. The Pavlidis Early Warning Test for Dyslexia promises early diagnosis and treatment of dyslexia and claims to have 90 per cent accuracy in detecting dyslexia in children as young as 5. There is also a Greek version of the Bangor Dyslexia Test available (Miles, 1993). However, the relatively small number of assessment tools available to teachers/practitioners to assist diagnosis, initial screening, or to indicate the progress achieved by those attending special classes has been another problem faced by practitioners in the area.

Remediation programmes vary as much in Greece as elsewhere. The main practice is increased exposure to reading/writing, although procedures do exist that have been developed primarily for the dyslexic child. For example, Maurommati (1995) uses pictures to connect key letters within words with the intended meaning or concept represented by that word. This latter technique may be particularly useful for a writing system in which the major problem for the learner is that different letters represent the same sound. For regular words, simple spelling–sound correspondence rules can be used to learn the correct spelling. However, for irregular (exception) words, where these rules do not apply, rote learning may be required. Providing a mnemonic which connects the correct representation of a sound (e.g., h, i and u for the 'ee' sound within a word), in a form which may be more easily recalled by the dyslexic child, may help the rote learning process, and provide a useful tool for the remedial or mainstream teacher struggling to explain those 'exceptions to the rule'.

REFERENCES

Maurommati, D. (1995) *The Establishment of a Programme to Cope with Dyslexia*. Athens. (In Greek.)

Miles, T.R. (1993) *Dyslexia: The Pattern of Difficulties*, 2nd edition. London: Whurr.

Ministry of Education and Religion (1994) *Information Manual of Special Education.* Athens: Department of Special Education Training. (In Greek.)

Porpodas, C.D. (1989) The phonological factor in reading and spelling of Greek. In P.G. Aaron and R.M. Joshi (eds), *Reading and Writing Disorders in Different Orthographic Systems.* Dordrecht: Kluwer Academic Publishers.

Porpodas, C.D. (1990) Processes used in children's reading and spelling of Greek words. In G. Th. Pavlidis (ed.), *Perspectives on Dyslexia.* Vol. 2 *Cognition, Language and Treatment.* Chichester: John Wiley.

ORGANIZATIONS

Ministry of Education and Religion
Department of Special Education
Ermou 15
101 85 Athens
Tel.: 0030-210-3231770
Tel.: 0030-210-3231811
Fax: 0030-210-3231770

Greek Dyslexia Association
Xenofontos 114
176 74 Kallithea
Athens
Tel.: 0030 210-9430787
Website: www.dyslexia.gr

Special Diagnostic. Research and Therapeutic Unit for the Child 'Spiros Doxiadis'
Gorgiou 6
Athens
Tel.: +30 210 9232347
Tel.: +30 210 9222666

Child Protection Centre
Michalinio
Akti Kountourioti 3
185 34 Pireaus
Tel.: +30 210 4172400

Psychological Centre of Xanthis
'Chrisa-Xanthis'
67100 Xanthi
Tel.: +30 2541 23755
Tel.: +30 2541 25182

Greek Society of Child's Psychological Health and Neuro-Psychatric
Semelis 34
115 28 Athens
Tel.: +30 210 7700570

Child's Hospital
Agia Sofia
Institute of Child's Health
Goudi
Athens
Tel.: +30 210 7794907
Tel.: +30 210 7715875

Audio-Psycho-Phonology Centre
79 Alexandras Avenue
Athens 11474
Tel.: +30 210 6411059

Psychiatric Health Centre
Ioulianou 18A Athens
Tel.: +30 210 3604929
Tel.: +30 210 3604972

Psychological Centre of Northern Greece
56701, Retziki
Thessaloniki
Tel.: +30 2310 93221

Centre of Psychiatric Health
Thessaloniki
Kaftatzoglou 36, 544639
Tel.: +30 2310 845130

Public Paediatric Neuropsychiatric Hospital
Ntaou Pentelis
19009 Rafina
Tel.: +30 294 23540

Centre for the Remediation of Dyslexic Children and Adults
Leoforou Marathonos 109
Pallini, T.K. 153 51
Tel.: +30 210 6667382

Medical and Paedagogical Centre of Neo Irakleio Attikis
Athens, Sokratous 32
N. Irakleio, T.K. 141 22
Tel.: +30 210 2816598

Neurolinguistic Institute
Athens
Greece
Email: ggnn@hol.gr

Ellenike Etairia Dyslexias
Iraklithon Street 41
Voula
177–73 Athens
Greece
Tel.: +30 1899 1817
Fax: +30 1960 4100

Student Resource Centre
University of La Verne
PO Box 51105
14510 Kifassia, Greece
Tel.: +30 1 6233 221
Email: src@laverne.edu.gr

CHAPTER AUTHORS

Maria Sp. Mazi
Kinopiastes
49084 Corfu
Greece
Tel.: +30 (0) 661 56356
Email: mazim@internet.gr

Styliani Nenopoulou
Department of Psychology
University of Surrey
Guildford
Surrey GU2 5XH. UK
Tel.: +44 (0) 1483 683977
Email: s.nenopoulou@surrey.ac.uk

John Everatt
Department of Psychology
University of Surrey
Guildford
Surrey GU2 5XH. UK
Tel.: +44 (0) 1483 686869
Email: j.everatt@surrey.ac.uk

DYSLEXIA IN HONG KONG

Suk-han Lee

HONG KONG: BACKGROUND

Schools

Of the almost 7 million inhabitants in Hong Kong, about one million attend school. Some 13 per cent of these students are enrolled in kindergartens, 68 per cent are enrolled in the nine-year basic education programmes (primary 1 to secondary 3) and 19 per cent in senior secondary education (secondary 4–7). In basic education, the average class size is 31.3 to 34.2 in the primary and 38.5 in the secondary programmes (EMB Key Statistics, 2003).

Languages

The language policy of the HKSAR government is to enable students and the population to be biliterate (i.e. in Chinese and English) and trilingual (i.e. in Cantonese, Putonghua and English). As Cantonese is only a spoken language, children have to learn the vocabulary and the grammar of standard Chinese when they learn to read and write. Having to learn more than one spoken and written language at such a young age inevitably poses challenges for those children who struggle with literacy acquisition.

The Education Reform

The long history of the competitive examination system in Hong Kong had led to many schools narrowing their curriculum to focus on 'examinable' aspects and on rote learning. In October 2000, the government launched the ambitious Education Reform with the vision of promoting students' ability to learn how to learn, to enhance their communication and literacy skills and develop multiple intelligence. Schools, supported by extra manpower and financial resources from the government, are urged to broaden their curriculum,

International Book of Dyslexia: A Guide to Practice and Resources. Edited by Ian Smythe, John Everatt and Robin Salter. ISBN 0-471-49646-4. © 2004 John Wiley & Sons, Ltd.

to develop diversified and effective assessment methods and to cater for the diverse learning needs of students so as to prevent failures in the education system.

LEGISLATION

The Code of Practice in Education (CoP – Equal Opportunity Commission, July 2001)

Pursuant to the Disability Discrimination Ordinance (DDO), the CoP informs schools and the public of the legal responsibilities of schools to ensure equal opportunities for students with disability. The document *Indicators of Inclusion*, to be published by the Education and Manpower Bureau (EMB), will provide a guide to schools on how to ensure that children with special needs, including those with dyslexia, are provided for.

DEFINITION

On the basic working definition of developmental dyslexia there is general consensus in Hong Kong. It refers to a child's severe and persistent difficulty in the acquisition of reading (word recognition) and dictation/spelling skills which is often unexpected in relation to age and other cognitive and academic abilities. Dyslexia has a neurological basis, and is not a result of global developmental disability, sensory impairment or brain damage, nor is it caused by environmental factors such as a lack of learning opportunity or severe emotional/behavioural disturbance. Current research evidence on dyslexia in Chinese points to a number of underlying cognitive deficits, including weakness in visual/orthographic skills, phonological awareness and phonological memory and automaticity. These children often also show problems in handwriting, organization and attention.

Terminology

While the term 'dyslexia' is commonly accepted in Hong Kong, organizations differ in their choice of terminology, often reflecting a difference in perspectives. The EMB has adopted the term 'specific learning difficulties'; the medical field, e.g. the Department of Health, as well as advocacy groups, prefer the term 'specific learning disabilities'; whereas other parties (e.g. the parents' group FOCUS) use the term 'specific learning differences'.

Diagnostic labelling

There is increasing awareness among educational psychologists of the limitations of the over-reliance on cut-off points of psychological tests for the 'black-and-white' diagnosis of dyslexia without taking into account instructional circumstances and the child's response to teaching. Problems of labelling arise particularly in cases where a child only shows some features of dyslexia but not all of them, or for whom there are other explanations for low literacy achievement. If persistence and severity in problems of literacy acquisition are a defining feature of dyslexia, assessment of a child's range of learning difficulties should be done over time in response to teaching. Front-line teachers should be trained to conduct assessment, interventions and monitoring of a child's progress at school, referring those children whose difficulties are most severe to the educational psychologist. Eligibility for remedial provisions or related services should be based on observed needs and not be dependent on the label of dyslexia.

Need for consensus

This alternative approach to the traditional 'specialist-assess-and-label' practice, in which the label of dyslexia seems to be more readily given, is perceived with much scepticism by advocacy groups who consider their demand for extra resources and accommodations to be justified by the label. There is a need for the different assessment agencies to arrive at some consensus on how and by whom assessment should be done and when the label of dyslexia is to be applied, otherwise confusion may arise. The crux of the matter, it seems, is whether a diagnostic label does or does not make a difference for the child to have access to the educational intervention which is needed.

Prevalence

No research data is available on prevalence rates. The establishment of prevalence is inherently difficult in view of the fact that individuals with dyslexia do not represent a homogeneous group, and that different prevalent rates may occur when different cut-off points are used. Nevertheless, it is interesting to note that figures available from the Education Department on the number of children assessed and classified by educational psychologists to have specific learning difficulties showed a rapid increase in recent years, e.g. from about 90 children in the 1992/93 school year to more than 900 children in 2001/2002. The publication of a teacher screening tool and an assessment tool for local psychologists, as well as the enhanced awareness among teachers, parents and the public might partly account for this increase.

IDENTIFICATION AND ASSESSMENT

Primary schools

The early identification and diagnostic assessment of dyslexia have been greatly facilitated by the publication of the *Hong Kong Specific Learning Difficulties Behaviour Checklist* for use by primary school teachers (October, 2000) and that of the *Hong Kong Test of Specific Learning Difficulties in Reading and Writing*, a Cantonese diagnostic battery for use by psychologists (August, 2000). Both instruments were developed by the Research Team on Specific Learning Difficulties jointly established by the University of Hong Kong, the Chinese University of Hong Kong and the EMB, with Dr Connie Ho as the project leader.

A Teachers' Guide and a Resource Pack with intervention strategies and worksheets have been developed by the EMB to enable teachers to provide timely remedial support to children subsequent to the screening using the Behaviour Checklist.

For the learning of English, a pilot project aimed at the early identification of primary one children at risk of reading difficulties is being conducted in ten primary schools in the

2002/03 school year, under the guidance of Professor Linda Siegel of UBC, Canada. Teachers will conduct assessment to identify those children with poorly developed phonological awareness and provide them with early intervention.

Secondary schools

Informal checklists are used in secondary schools for the identification of students suspected of having specific learning difficulties. Assessment is conducted by the psychologist through the use of standardized attainment tests, qualitative analysis of samples of work from the student and observational data of the type and extent of literacy difficulties. Assessment at secondary schools is hindered not only by the lack of standardized, normative instruments, but also by the fact that differential diagnosis may be complicated by accumulated backwardness resulting in low literacy attainment, secondary emotional or behavioural problems.

Assessment agencies

The bulk of the assessments is conducted by the two government departments, i.e. the Psychological Services under the EMB and the Child Assessment Centres and the Student Health Service under the Department of Health. Other assessment agencies include universities and psychologists in private practice.

INTERVENTION AND RESOURCES

Remedial services

Children with dyslexia are accommodated in mainstream schools in Hong Kong. Those requiring intensive remedial service receive it either at school or at off-site remedial centres operated by the EMB. Schools are encouraged to implement a whole school approach to support these children so that not only the remedial teacher but all teachers should be involved. A whole school policy specifying early identification and intervention of learning difficulties, monitoring of progress, assessment adaptations, curriculum differentiation, staff training on SEN management and parental involvement is the blueprint to replace the narrow definition of remedial service in the past.

Intervention strategies

Local research data has provided support that multi-sensory methods, training activities to enhance automaticity, paired reading and daily practice involving small targets are effective in helping dyslexic children to learn to read and dictate Chinese words. In addition, children are taught memory strategies such as 'Look, Say, Trace, Cover, Write, Check', chunking, visualization, using songs and other mnemonic devices, and study skills such as time management, colour coding and highlighters, self-questioning techniques, mindmapping, etc. Opportunities for success, which is essential in maintaining a child's motivation, must be provided.

Psycho-social support – centre-based

Learning support groups for parents are conducted by the EMB and the Child Assessment Centres. These aim at helping parents to understand the nature of their child's learning difficulties and to acquire some practical teaching strategies to enhance their learning. The Hong Kong Association for Specific Learning Disabilities, a parents' organization, runs a variety of activities for their members, both for parents and children.

School-based

Student Guidance personnel in primary and social workers in secondary schools organize activities such as talks and learning support programmes such as paired reading and study skills training for parents and students. An interesting model of psycho-social support, based on the 'Unique Mind School Programme' (developed by Marcia Stern of the Ackerman Institute for the Family in America to support learning disabled students and their families) is being tried out in a number of primary schools in Hong Kong.

Resources

The lack of commercial interest in producing resources for students with SEN has meant that resources for dyslexia are relatively limited and were developed almost exclusively by the EMB or by tertiary institutes with government funding. Resources developed so far can be grouped into (a) leaflets, resource pack and multimedia CDs for teachers, parents and the public, aimed at enhancing dyslexia awareness, promoting early recognition and teaching basic management skills; (b) multimedia CDs and resource teaching materials for teachers to use in the classroom, and (c) software learning programmes designed for use by the child to develop reading skills in Chinese and English. An overview of most of these resources can be seen on the website of Special Education Resource Centre (www.serc.emb.gov.hk).

ICT

Experiments with commercially available Cantonese voice recognition technology and the slow-down playback function of some tape-recorders to support children with phonological difficulties, as well as simplified methods of input in Chinese word-processing, all offer potential support to learning by dyslexic children in schools.

TEACHER TRAINING

Pre-service

Under the Education Reform, the Advisory Committee on Teacher Education and Qualifications (ACTEQ) is reviewing the content of teacher training courses to equip teachers more effectively to meet the diverse learning needs of students. This will hopefully enhance teacher preparation in the teaching of children with specific learning difficulties.

In-service

The EMB conducts many school-based workshops annually in order to promote the whole school approach in supporting children with specific learning difficulties. Territory-wide seminars and workshops are run by the ED as well as other organizations such as the Manulife Centre at the Polytechnic University and the Pathways Foundation, etc.

ADVOCACY GROUPS

The major dyslexia advocacy groups are the Specific Learning Disabilities Working Party of the Hong Kong Society of Child Neurology and Developmental Paediatrics (HKCNDP) led by paediatricians, and the Hong Kong Association of Specific Learning Disabilities (HKASLD), a parents association. Their efforts have led to much media coverage on dyslexia as well as support for their cause by some legislators. Other active parents associations include F.O.C.U.S. and the Dyslexia Association (Hong Kong) which hold monthly support meetings for their members.

EXAM PROVISIONS

The EMB has issued a set of guidelines and circular memoranda to schools on access to the curriculum and accommodations in internal assessments for the child with SEN, which includes specific learning difficulties. The Hong Kong Exam and Assessment Authority has set up a task group to develop a set of guidelines on special examination arrangements for children with specific learning difficulties.

THE WAY AHEAD

Children showing difficulties in the acquisition of literacy should be given timely help and the needed resource at school, with or without an official diagnostic label of dyslexia. At the systems level, the Education Reform, the Code of Practice in Education and the integrated whole school approach model all point to the role and the responsibility for schools to respond to the special learning needs of the child, through a broadened curriculum, diversified assessment methods and close collaboration between the teachers, parents and the student concerned.

The early recognition and early intervention for children with dyslexia and literacy difficulties depend on the teachers' awareness and their ability to teach to individual differences in the classroom, to monitor and review. Effective teacher training and development of teacher assessment tools and resources will be an important challenge to all teacher trainers.

ICT, including software and voice recognition technology, will create important learning support for the dyslexic Chinese child. The commercial sector needs to be stimulated to become a partner should we wish to develop such resources at a more rapid pace.

Research should inform practice, both in terms of a better understanding of the nature of dyslexia as well as the effectiveness of various forms of intervention.

NOTE

The opinions expressed in this chapter are those of the writer and do not represent those of the Hong Kong Education and Manpower Bureau.

ORGANIZATIONS

Special Education Resource Centre
Education and Manpower Burean
HKSAR Government
Website: serc.emb.gov.hk

Education City
HKSAR Government
Website: www.hkedcity.net

Equal Opportunity Commission
Website: www.eoc.org.hk

Research Team on Specific Learning Difficulties (Joint research team of the University of Hong Kong, Chinese University of Hong Kong and the EMB)
Website: hksld.psy.hku.hk

Manulife Centre for Specific Learning Disabilities
HK Polytechnic University
Website: nhs.polyu.edu.hk/mccsld/

Hong Kong Society of Child Neurology and Developmental Paediatrics
Website: www.fmshk.com.hk/hkcndp

Hong Kong Association for Specific Learning Disabilities (HKASLD)
Website: www.asld.org.hk

Pathways Foundation
Website: www.gsis.edu.hk/news_events/pathways

Dyslexia Association (Hong Kong)
Website: www.dyslexia.org.hk/

F.O.C.U.S.
Website: www.focus-hk.org

CHAPTER AUTHOR

Suk-han Lee
Educational Psychologist
C/O Education and Manpower Bureau
Psychological Services (Special Education) Section
18/F, Chinachem Tsuen Wan Plaza
457 Castle Peak Road
Tsuen Wan
Hong Kong Special Administration Region
China
Email: sukhanhk@netvigator.com

DYSLEXIA IN HUNGARY

Éva Gyarmathy and Emőke Vassné Kovács

INTRODUCTION

The first Hungarian expert in studying dyslexia was Ranschburg Pál (1916). He compared the reading speed of 100 normal and mentally disabled children and in 1928 he gave a summary of his findings. In his book he described the physiological, pathological, psychological and therapeutical aspects of the syndrome 'leghastenia' (as he called the reading difficulties). After a very long break, only in the 1960s was the work he started continued mainly by educational psychologists, who found reading difficulties as the background to school failure (Ligeti, 1967). Speech therapists (Meixner *et al.*, 1971; Kovács-Vass, 1980) had to face the fact that after correcting severe speech defects, children showed reading difficulties in school.

The close relation between linguistic development and the acquisition of literacy skills was realized in the 1960s, and as a consequence of this, dealing with dyslexic children became part of the speech therapy.

Since 1963 dyslexia (later also dyscalculia) has been part of the speech therapists' training. Trainee speech therapists learn the theory and the practice of it in the subject 'psychology'. They become familiar with some basic test methods: intelligence tests (WISC-R, SON) and other measures of different abilities (Bender, Frostig, Inizan), as well as with methods for developing basic abilities (Sindelar, 1994; Zsoldos, 1999). More subjects provide knowledge in psycholinguistic areas. Students learn assessment methods such as the Meixner (1993) vocabulary test, the Gósy (1995) GMP linguistic ability test, and the Kassai and Kovács (1992) verbal memory test. Trainee speech therapists gain experience in these methods in their school practice.

DYSLEXIA TERMINOLOGY

Since the 1990s educational policy-makers have understood the importance of the treatment of reading difficulties. The topic became part of teacher training.

International Book of Dyslexia: A Guide to Practice and Resources. Edited by Ian Smythe, John Everatt and Robin Salter. ISBN 0-471-49646-4. © 2004 John Wiley & Sons, Ltd.

Difficulties in reading, writing and/or counting are specific learning difficulties according to the official definition. Sarkady and Zsoldos (1987–88 and 1992–93) claimed:

> specific learning difficulty is to be identified if the learning achievement of the person is significantly below what is expected on the basis of the person's intelligence, and it has been developed on the ground of neurological deficit or malfunctioning, and shows a particular cognitive syndrome . . . It may be an associative syndrome of mental retardation, sensory impairment or speech defect.

Dyslexia was listed in the 'other retardation' category in a law in 1993. Those who show a particular cognitive psychological syndrome (disabilities in perception, speech production and linguistic abilities, malfunctioning attention and memory, difficulties in laterality and orientation) belong to this group.

The advantage of this law is that schools receive a higher range of financial support for the teaching of these children. The problem is that these children are labelled retarded, which is a rather degrading, and a discriminatory distinction. We have to add that to call dyslexic children retarded is not only derogatory, but also false, because behind the specific learning difficulties there is a diverse way of information processing, which can be very useful in appropriate situations (Gyarmathy, 1996).

Nevertheless, since this law came into effect the dyslexic person has had a better chance of receiving appropriate teaching. The other heterogeneous group where dyslexia has been included is 'linguistic disorders'. The reason for listing dyslexics in this group is the fact that logopaedical disorders are often associated with dyslexia (Gerebenné, 1995).

PREVENTION

Prevention gained greater and greater emphasis and became the most important part of the work and became logopaedical practice. Systematic screening was started in the nursery schools to discover the children 'at risk'. Many screening methods were adapted for this work. Later Hungarian psychologists, linguistics and speech therapists worked out methods for early identification of the signs of possible dyslexia. Many tests, including Bender, Frostig, Inizan, Sindelar, the Meixner vocabulary test, the Gósy GMP linguistic ability test, the Kassai and Kovács verbal memory test, were developed in this period.

The Dyslexia Prevention Test (DPT), developed by Marosits (1990), made possible the detailed examination of children. The test measures auditory discrimination, auditory memory, spatial orientation, visuality, sense of rhyming, fine movement and drawing abilities. Results help to decide what kind of specialist – ophthalmologist, audiologist, ear, nose and throat specialist, teacher of special needs, psychologist or neurologist – has to be involved to give appropriate support.

Another route in the prevention of dyslexia was created by educational psychologists. Porkolábné Balogh (1992) and Gyarmathy (1991) devised preventive sensori-motor skills improving programmes for nursery and primary schools. The concept was based on the fact that the sensitive period of the sensori-motor skills is between the age of 3 and 6. The basic abilities for the literacy skills develop powerfully, and can be strengthened effectively during that period. Exercises and games that develop sensori-motor skills can be built into the everyday life of the nursery and used regularly in the first years in the primary school.

As the result of these programmes children became more prepared for school and more severe problems were identified early. Children were sent to specialists or treated in the nursery in a small remediation group. Unfortunately these methods have not spread because they need preparatory training and some extra work. Nursery schools are crowded and teachers are overburdened with work.

THERAPIES

In the past ten years more teaching and therapeutical materials have been developed for dyslexics of different ages in Hungary, thanks to the support of foundations (Kovács and Szebényi-Torda, 1992; Marosits, 1994; Vannay, 1995, Rosta, 1996; Vekerdi, 1998). The new materials gave the methodological background for the therapeutical work after the constitutional changes.

To give correct support and service attitudes had to be changed. Formerly, dyslexia was recognized mostly in school when the child failed. We know those dyslexic disorders that lead to literacy problems, and it is possible to start early, many-sided, intensive treatment and often individual education plans are used.

In many cases the treatment has not provided sufficient support. That led to the formation of logopaedical nursery groups and later whole logopaedical nursery schools. These nursery schools can offer some children a tolerant educational environment, which can promote the development of abilities as well as the personality of the children. The therapy is disability specific and children get support to develop basic skills, sensori-motor, communicational and linguistic skills. The prevention of dyslexia and dyscalculia is built on these treatments. About 50 per cent of the children suffering from severe language disorders receive support that way.

Depending on the severity of the disorder, children can be integrated into the normal schools, or they continue learning in special logopaedical classes. There are increasing numbers of classes for these children, but they are unable to satisfy the increasing demand.

In a class for dyslexic children the maximum of 15 pupils provides the optimal educational situation, and also make individual education possible. There is no written homework, all the tasks that involve writing are solved in the school. There is graphomotor training and speech therapy every day.

There are more and more private and foundation schools for children with specific learning difficulties. These schools provide small group education, individual plans and special training. The instruction is adapted to the abilities and needs of the children. Thus, increasing numbers of severe dyslexic children receive a secondary education and achieve the certificate of final examination.

INTEGRATION

The final aim of the treatment of dyslexic individuals is the earliest possible social integration. The route and the phases of the integration depend mainly on the age, on the severity of the disturbance and on the presence of other associated deficits. The solution is usually individual.

The re-education of primary schoolchildren aims to give a base for writing and reading through the development of the basic skills and the metalinguistic abilities, and to raise the level of reading by the increase in the child's vocabulary.

The most frequent syndromes in the secondary school are disturbances of the visual perception, short-term memory deficits and difficulties in comprehension. The epiphenomena such as low self-esteem, aggression or withdrawal cause at least as much of a problem as the linguistic disabilities. There is more and more software for dyslexics to develop their abilities through play, which makes the exercises more interesting and acceptable, but this hardly helps to avoid the everyday failure in the classrooms.

Unfortunately, the average teacher is not aware of the problems of dyslexic children and youngsters. It is still characteristic that dyslexic children are considered to be lazy or mentally disabled. Many teachers are unable to accept that a person can be intelligent and yet unable to read.

Current teaching methods do not help dyslexic children in their studies. The traditional instruction causes difficulties for these students in comprehension – they simply cannot follow the teacher's speech. There is written homework every day, and the study books contain lengthy text, which is a disaster for the dyslexic child.

TEACHER TRAINING

One of the most important steps for the provision of dyslexic individuals is to train teachers by giving them a thorough knowledge and understanding of dyslexia, with appropriate methods for teaching dyslexic children.

Trainee teachers of the handicapped get much information, knowledge and practice in specific learning difficulties. However, average teachers in the comprehensive schools hardly ever hear about dyslexia during their training.

Fortunately, there are more and more official courses on this topic for teachers in Hungary. These courses give expertise mostly in linguistic areas. However, there are programmes for the development of basic abilities, as well. Teachers are taught to assess children and lead special programmes for them.

LAWS

Dyslexic children were listed as handicapped students by an educational law in 1993. It means that schools receive extra financial support for the rehabilitation of these children. That way individual programmes and education in small classes became attainable for learning disabled children.

In accordance with the needs of the student, the headteacher can exempt the child with specific learning difficulties from a problematic subject. Similarly, these students are allowed to choose another subject instead of the problematic one for the final examination in the Hungarian secondary school.

Unfortunately, it became a common custom to exempt dyslexics from learning foreign languages. It means that these students are not obliged to attend the language lessons. As a result of this procedure, dyslexic children are unable to speak foreign languages, which is very disadvantageous to their future prospects considering that Hungarian is a rather rarely used language in the world. Foreign languages should be taught differently for dyslexic students and their achievement should be assessed by using more appropriate methods.

Since 1993, there has also been a specialist secondary school for dyslexics; however, the methods used in this school are only partly adequate for the abilities of dyslexic students. Though there is great emphasis on computers and using multimedia, the methods used in the traditional subjects are the traditional old methods.

FUTURE OUTLOOK

Since the concept of dyslexia has been officially accepted and much more support has been given to solve the problem, Hungarian experts must create a more coherent system for the treatment of dyslexia. Specialists working in different fields should communicate with each other, and work out a comprehensive test to measure the abilities of dyslexics distinctively, to identify the child's deficiencies and strengths in order to understand its needs.

As there are more suitable teaching and learning methods for dyslexic students, the next task is to disseminate and popularize their use in the comprehensive schools and in schools and classes for children with specific learning difficulties. This can be accomplished only if these methods are taught in the teacher training colleges, and teachers accept changes in the traditional instruction.

REFERENCES

Gerebenné Várbíró, K. (1995) Szempontok a nyelvi fejlődés zavarának értelmezéséhez. [Considerations on the interpretation of disturbances of linguistic development.] In *Fejlödési diszfázia.* BGGYTF szerk.: Gerebenné dr. Várbíró K., Budapest.

Gósy, M. (1995) *GMP Diagnosztika.* Budapest: Nikol.

Gyarmathy, É. (1991) Játékkatalógus: tanulási zavarokkal küzdő gyerekek. [Collection of games for children with specific learning difficulties.] In P. Balogh K., *Iskolapszichológia,* 20. ELTE, Budapest.

Gyarmathy, É. (1996) Tanulási zavarokkal küzdő tehetséges gyerekek azonosítása. [Identification of gifted children with specific learning difficulties.] PhD thesis. Debrecen: Kossuth Lajos Tudományegyetem.

Kassai, I. and Kovács, E. (1992) A nyelvi készségek és a diszlexia kapcsolatáról. [Linguistic skills and dyslexia.] *Fejlesztő Pedagógia* 3–4, 54–56.

Kovács, Á., Szebényi, É. and Torda, Á. (1992) *Mondd ki, írd le, törd a fejed!* [Say, write and think!] Budapest: Nemzeti Tankönyvkiadó.

Kovács-Vass, E. (1980) *Verbal Communication as the Prerequisite of the Development of Communication in Writing. Communication and Handicap Report of EASE 80.* The Finnish Association for Special Education.

Ligeti, R. (1967) Gyermekek olvasászavarai. [Children's reading disorders.] *Pszichológia a gyakorlatban IX.* Budapest: Akadémiai Kiadó.

Marosits, A. (1990) *Diszlexia Prevenciós Tesztcsomag (DPT).* Budapest: Logopress.

Marosits, A. (1994) *Betűző.* [Speller] Logopédiai GMK.

Meixner, I. (1993) *A dyslexia prevenció, reedukáció módszere.* [Method of dyslexia prevention and reeducation.] Budapest: BGGYTF.

Meixner, I., Kovács, T. and Vekerdi, Zs. (1971) *Módszertani közlemények I.* [Methodology.] Debrecen: Magyar Pedagógiai Társaság.

Porkolábné Balogh, K. (1992) *Kudarc nélkül az iskolába.* [Without failure in the school.] Budapest: Alex-Typo.

Ranschburg, P. (1916) *Die Leseschwäche /Legasthenie/ und Rechnenschwäche /Arithmasthenie/ der Schulkinder im Lichte des Experimentes.* Berlin.

Sarkady, K. and Zsoldos, M. (1992–93) Koncepcionális kérdések a tanulási zavar fogalom körül. [Conceptual issues on the notion of specific learning difficulties.] *Magyar Pszichológiai Szemle*, 18–19 (3–4), 259–270.

Sindelar, B. (1994) *Teilleistungsschwächen.* Vienna: Eigenverlag.

Vannay, J. (1995) *Szófejtő, szórejtő.* [Logographs.] Budapest: Logopédiai GMK.

Vekerdi, I. (1998) Nyelvi játékok az óvodában. [Linguistic games in the nursery.] *Beszédgyógyítás*, 2, 15–77.

Zsoldos, M. (1999) A tanulási és magatartási zavarok kognitív terápiája – A Sindelar-program. [Cognitive therapy of the learning and behavioural disturbances – The Sindelar programme.] *Új Pedagógiai Szemle*, XLIX (1), 70–77.

ORGANIZATIONS

Diszlexiás Gyermekekért Egyesület
Nemzetkozi Konferencia Kozpoint,
1114 Vilanyi Ut 11-13
Budapest
Hungary
Tel.: +36 1 30605 84
Email: mate@ludens.elte.hu

Startdyslexia, Eszékutca 5
1114 Budapest
Hungary
Email: hegedusfam@axelero.hu

Magyar Diszlexia Oldalak
Website: www.diszlexia.hu

CHAPTER AUTHORS

Éva Gyarmathy and Emőke Vassné Kovács
Magyar Tudományos Akadémia
Pszichológiai Kutatóintézet
Cím: H-1132 Budapest
Victor Hugo u. 18-22.
Tel.: 361-279-6000
Email: gyarme@mtapi.hu

DYSLEXIA IN INDIA

Philip John, Susan K. George and Anu B. Mampilli

PARADIGM SHIFT: FROM THE HEALTH SECTOR TO EDUCATION

A national response to the problem of Learning Disorders (LD) including dyslexia is lacking in India. Barriers to care include lack of awareness among government agencies, policy-makers of Education Boards, teachers and parents. Primary care physicians, pediatricians and even psychiatrists are not well enough equipped to objectively evaluate all the causes of Poor School Performance (PSP) in a child. There are, therefore, monumental issues in both the Health and Education Sectors in grappling with this silent handicap affecting about 10 per cent of school children (Philip et al., 2001).

The historical background of the evolution of the concept of dyslexia placed it, unfortunately, under the rubric of the Health Sector. But the sheer force of numbers of children afflicted by this malady persuades us to shift and move this responsibility to the mainstream Education infrastructure. What is required then is to provide trained 'Educational Diagnosticians' to create a 'National Action Plan' in the educational sector for holistic, comprehensive and reasonably uniform assessment and remediation of Learning Disorders and co-morbid conditions.

INDIA: BACKGROUND

India presents imponderable issues in this area. The major hurdle is our country's multilingual pluralism and linguistic diversity. India's 1,000 million people use at least 1,600 mother tongues and the country boasts 20 recognized languages. These regional languages evolved from diverse language families, mainly the Aryan in North India and the Dravidian in the South. The Indian Constitution recognizes Hindi as the official language and English as the legislative and judicial language. Britain's colonial rule unified the diverse ethnic elements through the English language which is a sort of lingua franca. Every school

International Book of Dyslexia: A Guide to Practice and Resources. Edited by Ian Smythe, John Everatt and Robin Salter. ISBN 0-471-49646-4. © 2004 John Wiley & Sons, Ltd.

child now is faced with this astounding complexity – having to speak one language at home and study a minimum of three languages in school, including Hindi and English.

To complicate matters further, there are several School Education Boards – the Central Board of Secondary Education (CBSE) and the All India Council for School Examination (AICSE). These have regulations common to the entire country and their schools abroad, while each of the 28 States and 7 Union Territories has independent Examination Boards with regulations which apply only to those territories. The medium of instruction may be chosen – English, Hindi or a regional language.

It is, nevertheless, mandatory that the child learns at least three languages starting even at the primary level. The plethora of problems for a dyslexic child is compounded by such a system of multilingual exposure. In our experience at Cochin, most of the dyslexic children are found to be worse in oriental languages than in English. This may be due to their complex script or phoneme–grapheme correspondence; however, this needs further validation (George, 1999). As great a hurdle is the current educational system and examinations which rely heavily (and sometimes exclusively) on written performance.

LEGISLATION AND POLICIES

In spite of overwhelming evidence of Learning Disorders being Special Educational Needs (SEN), the Persons with Disabilities Act (PWD Act) was passed by the Indian Parliament in 1995 without including LD. Nor does the Rehabilitation Council of India Act recognize dyslexia as a disability, in spite of expert committee recommendations and vociferous advocacy by non-governmental organizations, thus depriving dyslexic children of their rightful provisions for rehabilitation.

However, the country has made significant strides in the areas of teacher sensitization and provisions for dyslexic children through the determined efforts of Educational Boards. The CBSE has taken pioneering steps by organizing Teacher Training/Orientation Programmes, by publishing handbooks for teachers on causes and remediation of Poor School Performance (PSP), etc. The State Boards are following suit, though tardily. The current educational policy stresses the concept of inclusive education, advocating that children with Special Needs (SEN) use the mainstream educational infrastructure.

EXAMINATION AND CURRICULUM PROVISIONS

In spite of policy-makers and teachers obstinately maintaining that dyslexia is only a problem of pushy parents or a fantasy of researchers, bold initiatives by various Examination Boards, especially CBSE, have come as a boon to these differently-abled children.

Curriculum provisions are being put in place to allow dyslexic children to choose alternatives such as Arts, Music, Home Science or Information Technology, but these policies are ill-understood by many school administrators; eligibility for provisions is not uniform across the various Boards either.

Constructing a uniform national policy to assess and certify eligibility for provisions in examinations has become a contentious issue. A structured, multidisciplinary team evaluation along with the school report is being advocated to ensure transparency. Dyslexic children so certified are currently allowed extra time, the use of calculators, the use of an amanuensis, and consideration of content against spellings in their examinations.

The National Open School (NOS) curriculum devised for the academically and socially disadvantaged children allows private registrations for Board examinations and choice of vocational courses such as IT, carpentry, printing, horticulture, etc. instead of languages. These students can appear for the final examinations in instalments if they so decide. The curriculum is validated as equivalent to the other Boards across the country.

IDENTIFICATION: TEACHER AS DIAGNOSTICIAN AND THERAPIST

There are no reliable data about remedial services available across the country; there is certainly no uniformity in the diagnostic criteria or types of remedial services provided (Ramaa, 1992). The national picture of access to services is quite uneven, with agencies and specialists being available mostly in the urban areas alone. This is where a paradigm shift is called for, to deal with the enormous number of children needing services. Some 20–25 per cent of children in every class score 'poor marks'. Therefore, the best place to identify dyslexia is the classroom itself.

Our strategy has been path-breaking, to consider 'poor marks' as a symptom (Philip *et al.*, 2001). Then, the class teacher is trained as a 'therapist' to use a simple and brief algorithm to 'diagnose' the various causes in the particular child which have led to Poor School Performance (PSP). These causes include: (1) hearing or visual deficits; (2) subnormal intelligence (IQ); (3) Learning Disorders including dyslexia; (4) Attention Deficit Disorders; and (5) emotional/behaviour disorders. Teachers, through brief structured sensitization, can thus be easily empowered to become 'Educational Diagnosticians'.

The causes of PSP include a synthesis of educational, social, psychological and neurological factors. Therefore, a restricted Educational model without a multidisciplinary, multiaxial perspective may only see dyslexia in isolation. Such an evaluation can blind the professional to the presence of co-existing neurodevelopmental, environmental or behavioural disorders in the dyslexic child. Our 'Diagnostic Approach' overcomes this problem effectively, and creates a holistic perspective.

The CBSE has recognized the potential of this approach. It has been training its teachers using a Handbook prepared by the authors of this chapter to develop a national resources organization and to achieve uniformity in the identification and management of Poor School Performance.

CO-MORBID DISORDERS: THE MULTIDISCIPLINARY APPROACH

Poor School Performance (PSP) evaluated at our centre at Cochin, South India, yielded very useful information. Of 1,310 cases of PSP in a two-year period, 65.8 per cent were diagnosed with Learning Disorders (LD). Among them 62.7 per cent had significant and diagnosable psychological co-morbidity. Attention deficit hyperactivity disorders, obsessive compulsive disorders, oppositional defiant/conduct disorders, Tourette's disorder, anxiety, school phobia and depression are the prominent co-morbid disorders identified.

What is more significant is that in 31 per cent of these children, developmental communication disorders (speech and language disorders) and developmental co-ordination disorders (motor skill disorders) were also detected. We are now cognizant of this pattern and tend to see them – linguistic, cognitive and motor developmental disorders – as occurring in a spectrum.

RESULTS FROM THE COCHIN EXPERIENCE

Our emerging data give clear messages:

1 In view of multiaxial deficits in children with LD, any resource centre should adopt a multidisciplinary 'diagnostic' approach to Poor School Performance (PSP).
2 Considering the types of co-morbidity, the multidisciplinary team under one roof must consist of special educators, psychologists, speech and language pathologists, professional social workers trained in LD, and a psychiatrist.
3 The yield from such an evaluation of the LD child is a comprehensive profile of his academic skill deficits as well as strengths and potential, discrepancy factor, expressive and receptive language and speech deficits, attention, activity, and behaviour problems as well as family and school support systems. This profile is used to prepare his Individualized Education Programme (IEP).
4 LD co-exists with clinical psychiatric disorders to be routinely looked for – ADHD, anxiety and phobic disorders, tics and obsessive disorders, depressive disorders, oppositional defiant or conduct disorders, etc. as well as neurodevelopmental deficits in language and motor skills.
5 LD predisposes an otherwise healthy child to the development of psychological disorders.
6 Presence of LD predicts a more guarded prognosis in a child with co-existing psychological disorder.
7 Remediation of LD becomes holistic and meaningful only when related co-morbid disorders are addressed concurrently. Ideal comprehensive remedial strategies involve remediation of academic skill deficits, psychological support strategies and, in many cases, sagacious use of pharmacological intervention with family support.

CONCLUSION

Resource centres must be manned by a relevant multidisciplinary team to offer a comprehensive management programme for each referred child with Poor School Performance.

In such a programme, academic assistance and remediation are not enough; the mental health issues of all academically-challenged children are to be concurrently addressed. Making it mandatory for each school to inform and train its classroom teachers as well as to set up resource rooms with special educators for the differently-abled children should be the ambitious, yet feasible, goal.

The core strategy, however, in the immediate identification and remediation of learning disorders including dyslexia, lies in empowering mainstream Teachers to become 'Educational Diagnosticians' – a paradigmatic shift from the health rubric to the educational sector.

REFERENCES

Philip, J. (1997) Learning disabilities: From health to education. Paper presented at National Conference on LD, Chennai, India.

Philip, J. (2002) Co morbid psychological disorders in LD Children, in P. Karanth (ed.), *Learning Disabilities: A Multidisciplinary Perspective*. London: Sage Publications.

Philip, J., George, S.K. and Mampilli, A.B. (2001) *Handbook on Poor School Performance*. Delhi: Central Board of Secondary Education.

Ramaa, S. (1992) *Package on LD*. Mysore: National Council of Educational Research and Training.

George, S.K. (1999) Learning disabilities in the Indian context: Current issues in management. Paper presented at National Seminar on LD, Osmania University, Hyderabad, India.

ORGANIZATIONS

G. Balasubramanian
Director of Academics
CBSE
New Delhi-110092

Peejay's Child Guidance Clinic (CGC)
Valanjambalam
Cochin 682 016
Kerala
India

Prathiba S. Karanth
Bangalore Institute of Institute of Speech and Hearing
Hennur Road
Bangalore
India

Lalitha Ramanujan
58 New Avadi Road
Kilpauk
Chennai 600 010
India

Nirmala Pandit
Madras Dyslexia Association
10/1 Sambasivam Street
T. Nagar
Chennai 600 017
India

Onita Nakra
Special Education Centre
D6/1 Vasanth Vihar
New Delhi 110057
India

Rukmini Krishnaswamy, 31,
5th Cross, 5th Main
Indira Nagar Stage I
Bangalore 560 038
India

S. Ramaa
Department of Special Education
Regional College of Education
Mysore 570 006
India

Smriti Swaroop
Department of Special Education
SNDT Women's University
Juhu Road
Mumbai 400 049
India

Sunita Sodhi
Educare Charitable Trust
M-2m Hauz Khas
New Delhi 110 048
India

Vinita Pandit
Maharashtra Dyslexia Association
303 Jharna
Dr Ambedkar Road
Khar (West)
Mumbai 400 052
India

CHAPTER AUTHORS

Philip John
Peejay's Polyclinic and EEG Labs
Valanjambalam
Cochin 682 016
Kerala
India
Tel.: 0484 235 7598/0484 2 36 6293
Email: peejaycl@hotmail.com

Susan K. George and Anu B. Mampilli
Peejay's Child Guidance Clinic (CGC)
Valanjambalam
Cochin 682 016
Kerala
India
Tel.: 0484 2 35 7388
Email: sussgorg@yahoo.com

DYSLEXIA IN IRAN

L.G. Tehrani

PERSIAN ORTHOGRAPHY

Persian (Farsi) has adopted the Arabic alphabet with some modifications. The script consists of a total of 32 characters comprising 28 Arabic characters with an additional four representing Persian phonemes that are not found in Arabic (see Figure 1).

Four important features of the Persian writing system should be noted. The shape, the position (initial, medial and final) of the characters, the number of dots as well as their position (above or below) are important for the identification of each grapheme (examples are given in Figure 2).

With respect to shape, the letters are divided into two groups. One group is called connectors and the other non-connectors. Twenty-five of the 32 characters are considered connectors, because they are connected to the neighbouring grapheme (right or left) when they appear in the word.

The grapheme–phoneme correspondence of the Persian writing system is complicated by the borrowed nature of the alphabet. Only 16 of the characters represent one single phoneme in each case. In the remainder of the cases, some sort of discrepancy exists between the sound and its representing grapheme. For example, a single phoneme may be represented by four different characters. In Arabic, each character would have its own phoneme, but because these phonemes do not exist in the Persian language, they are used to represent the Persian phoneme that is most similar to their Arabic counterpart. Examples can be found in Figure 3.

Another major source of difficulty is due to the style of representation of vowels. In most instances there is no grapheme representation for the short vowels, which are represented by diacritics (see examples in Figure 4).

Long vowels, on the other hand, are represented by three of the 32 characters in the alphabet.

International Book of Dyslexia: A Guide to Practice and Resources. Edited by Ian Smythe, John Everatt and Robin Salter. ISBN 0-471-49646-4. © 2004 John Wiley & Sons, Ltd.

/P/ پ   /č/ چ   /ž/ ژ   /g/ گ

FIGURE 1   Four characters representing Persian phonemes that are not found in Arabic

M	Final	Medial	Initial
	م	ـمـ	مـ
	دیدم	فهمید	مرد
	I saw	He/She understood	Man
	پ	ت	ب
	/P/	/T/	/B/

FIGURE 2   Examples of Persian characters representing initial, medial and final positions

/Z/	ظ	ض	ذ	ز
	ظهر	مریض	ذغال	زهره
	/zohr/	/mariz/	/zogal/	/zohre/

FIGURE 3   Examples of inconsistencies between characters and sounds in the Persian alphabet

/a/ ◌َ   ;   /Ma/ مَ

/e/ ◌ِ   ;   /Me/ مِ

/o/ ◌ُ   ;   /Mo/ مُ

FIGURE 4   Examples of diacritical marks used to represent short vowels in Persian

READING AND WRITING DIFFICULTIES IN PERSIAN

The above features of the script lead to reading being relatively easier than spelling (dictation) in Persian. The method used in Iran to teach literacy skills is based on the phonic method and emphasizes the relationship between characters and speech sounds. Therefore, as soon as the student becomes familiar with the alphabet, they are able to read most Farsi words. However, there are some common mistakes in every student's reading at the early stages of acquisition. These include (1) difficulties in reading new words that do not make sense to them without diacritics; (2) problems reading words that look like one another; and (3) errors related to verb inflection – even though through the sentence structure the student can guess the correct verb inflection, differences between spoken and written form of inflection increase this kind of misreading.

Although reading words including Arabic letters can be a little confusing for Persian-speaking children, it is much easier than spelling them in dictation. In particular, the Persian language beginner reader often has difficulty in writing homophones. Some common mistakes, which are seen more often in the writing of dyslexics and poor readers than normal achieving students, are (1) decreasing or increasing connected symbols, duplication and dots; (2) attachment or detachment of one letter to another; and (3) lack of diacritic symbols, increasing diacritics, word and letter omission, etc. All these mistakes are individualized and need special attention.

THE IRANIAN SCHOOL SYSTEM

There are five years of education at primary school in Iran. This is followed by secondary school that consists of a further three academic years. High school comprises four more years during which the students study those subjects that are academic of interest to them. In recent years, some schools have accepted students one year prior to entry to primary school. The usual age of entry to primary school is six. This preparatory year would, therefore, start with children who are five years old. Once formal schooling is started, all children receive the same instruction regardless of whether they have been in a preparatory year or not.

AWARENESS AND ASSESSMENT

There is a problem with awareness of specific learning difficulties in Iran. A high percentage of Iranian people label dyslexic children as mentally retarded and there is a lack of explicit knowledge of literacy problems. However, the increase in research in this area (for example, see Amini, 1997), as well as the increase in the numbers of graduating psychologist and speech therapists, have helped in the raising of public awareness of learning difficulties.

The identification of the existence of hearing, speech or visual problems is possible through primary screening tests that any child would have to do before entering school. However, there is no recognized way to diagnose dyslexic children prior to them finishing first grade. At this point, any child who shows difficulty learning to read letters, words and text, as well as having difficulties in spelling Persian letters and words properly, has been labelled as dyslexic. Given the lack of an explicit definition of dyslexia and clear criteria to evaluate children with learning difficulties, it is not clear whether further evaluation by psychometric methods and speech therapy examinations will reduce the number of children called dyslexic. One to 3 per cent of the pupils between 8 and 11 years old have been recognized as dyslexic children in Tehran, the capital of Iran. However, in some reported research this incidence increases to 5.5 per cent because poor and slow readers were counted as dyslexics as well (see Danekar, 1993). An understanding of the factors that lead to reading and writing difficulties among Persian-speaking children (see reports by Shirazi, 1995; Tehrani Gholami, 1996) should improve estimates of incidence.

Primary school teachers and speech therapists in major cities usually perform reading and writing assessments. Although there is no standard Persian reading and writing tests, informal procedures have been developed. Intensive phonological training at the start of the first grade enables teachers to recognize those students who have severe to mild literacy learning problems. In the following months, if the child shows continued difficulty in reading and writing, then the teachers can pay special attention to these dyslexic children.

SPECIAL TRAINING AND SPECIAL SCHOOLS

Since 1970, there have been specially trained teachers for those children who are mentally retarded in the Iranian education system. However, the Advanced Studies and Sciences Ministry established a four-year programme to train special teachers in 1981. Those who graduate from this programme have a high level of knowledge of psychology, psychometrics, behaviour therapy, and speech and language sciences. This degree enabled teachers to diagnose and intervene earlier.

Recently two supportive educational centres have been established in Tehran for those children who are studying in ordinary schools and suffering from dyslexia. These procedures provide for two to three extra lessons per week so that the dyslexic child can keep up with the rest of the children in their year group. Additionally, there are a number of private special schools dedicated to teaching dyslexic children. Their programmes cover the school curriculum as well as speech and behaviour therapy.

Unfortunately, there are no supporting programmes at secondary and high school levels for dyslexic children. Any difficulties that have not been overcome by the end of primary education, or new areas of difficulties, may go unassessed and lead to further educational difficulties.

REFERENCES

Amini, M. (1997) *Differences between Normal and Dyslexic Children in Reading and Writing Persian Texts.* Tehran: College of Rehabilitation Sciences.

Danekar, M. (1993) *Rate of Dyslexic Children in Iranian Schools.* Tehran: Education Department, University of Tehran.

Shirazi, T.S. (1996) *Phonological Awareness as an Important Predictor of Reading Acquisition in Persian-speaking Children.* Tehran: University of Rehabilitation and Social Welfare.

Tehrani Gholami, L. (1995) *Reading and Writing Difficulties in Persian-language Children.* Tehran: University of Rehabilitation and Social Welfare.

CHAPTER AUTHOR

L.G. Tehrani
University of Surrey
Guildford GU2 7XH
Surrey
Email: Lgtehrani@hotmail.com

DYSLEXIA IN IRELAND

Anne Hughes

REPORT OF TASK FORCE ON DYSLEXIA – 2001

In September 2000 the then Minister for Education and Science, Dr Michael Woods, set up a Task Force on Dyslexia. Members of the Task Force included teachers, psychologists, officials of the Department of Education and Science and other interested professionals. Alan Sayles, Education Consultant to the Dyslexia Association of Ireland and President of the European Dyslexia Association was a member. Over 1,400 individuals and organizations made written or verbal submissions. The Task Force reviewed the current range of educational provision and support for children with dyslexia, assessed its adequacy and made 61 recommendations.

The Report provided a useful definition of specific learning difficulty, advised individualization of provision for students and underlined the need for continuing professional development for teachers at all levels. The Report also pointed to the need for parents/guardians to be involved in multi-disciplinary teams to assess and review their children's needs, and noted the urgent need for information provision. This widely welcomed and long-awaited Report was comprehensive and, if its recommendations are implemented, will be a blueprint for the equitable and effective management of dyslexia in the Irish educational system.

HISTORICAL CONTEXT

The Report of the Task Force is the most positive development in the 30-year history of dyslexia in Ireland. This has in many ways been an inglorious history, marred for many years by disagreements over terminology, which often distracted from the necessary work in hand. Remedial education in its broadest sense did not come to the Republic of Ireland until the mid-1960s. The task of remedial teachers was to provide support for pupils who

International Book of Dyslexia: A Guide to Practice and Resources. Edited by Ian Smythe, John Everatt and Robin Salter. ISBN 0-471-49646-4. © 2004 John Wiley & Sons, Ltd.

were identified by class teachers as falling behind their peers, but who did not meet the criteria for admission to a special school. Psycho-educational assessment was very difficult to obtain and for the most part was provided for pupils who exhibited a general learning difficulty and for whom placement in a special school was considered appropriate. This assessment was available only from clinical psychologists working with the Department of Health. The concept of specific reading difficulty was relatively unknown. Anecdotal evidence from adults indicates that mis-diagnosed specific reading problems resulted in the placement of some pupils with average intelligence in special schools.

It was not until the 1970s that the term dyslexia came to be applied in cases of reading difficulty. This was almost entirely due to the work of the newly formed Dyslexia Association of Ireland. This voluntary organization was set up by parents Noelle Cleary and Eileen Dardis, supported by a small group of teachers. The aims of the founding group were to promote public awareness of dyslexia; to lobby the government for state provision for children with dyslexia; and in the interim to provide extra-curricular classes for reading.

One of the main difficulties faced by the Association in its early years was that of definition. The term 'dyslexia' was used by the Association, but was dismissed as vague and unscientific by many teachers, psychologists and, crucially, the Department of Education. Many futile battles were fought over whether such a condition as 'dyslexia' existed. Valuable time was wasted in debating this issue with the Department, while the real issue of service provision was neglected. As the Association was by then offering help to children with attention deficit disorder, hyperactivity, dyspraxia and mild language disorders, it was agreed to change the name to ACLD (The Association for Children and Adults with Learning Disabilities) in 1986. It was hoped that this would remove at least one area of contention and allow efforts to be concentrated on dealing with the problem. Working relations with the Department of Education improved and over the years a constructive partnership developed. The Department now provides a small grant each year to assist the work of the Association.

The Association reverted to its original name The Dyslexia Association of Ireland in October 2000. By a nice irony the change of name was formally launched by the Minister for Education and Science, Dr Woods, who declared that 'dyslexia' was his preferred term.

IDENTIFICATION AND SUPPORT

While the current educational provision for students with dyslexia in Ireland is far from ideal, it has improved vastly over the past decade. In the 1980s there were only four special reading schools at primary level, three in Dublin and one in Cork. Outside of the large cities there was very little help available. Now, special reading units within primary schools have been established and this appears to be the preferred format for the future. While the impetus for reading units originally came from parents, school principals are now requesting such classes and this is a very welcome development. These classes, with an 11 : 1 pupil teacher ratio are partially integrated into the mainstream. Increasing numbers of remedial and resource teachers are being employed, particularly at primary level. Departmental figures state that over 90 per cent of all state primary schools have access to a Learning Support teacher. This does not mean that all children with specific reading problems receive remedial help as pupils attending learning support teachers must be reading at or below the 10th percentile. Access to resource teachers is restricted to those children achieving at the 2nd percentile or lower, on standardized reading tests.

The National Educational Psychological Service (NEPS) was established in 1999 and by January 2002 it employed 120 psychologists. The target figure of 200 educational psychologists is expected to be reached by 2004. While a major objective of NEPS is to provide psycho-educational assessment for children with learning difficulties, waiting lists are still very long – up to two years or more and many parents still have to seek private assessment. However, the service now exists and it will expand.

There is no nationally applied screening test for early detection of specific reading difficulty. Some schools do use standardized screening checklists, but a recent report on Remedial Education in Irish Primary Schools (1998) reported that teacher observation was the most common procedure used to identify reading difficulty. The report also showed that most teachers do not fully understand dyslexia and are not trained to recognize or manage the condition. This is why adequate training at pre-service level is such a large issue.

A survey of parent members of the Dyslexia Association recently revealed that 73 per cent of respondents were not satisfied with the help their child received in school, 69 per cent felt that the teachers encountered by their children were not sufficiently aware of the needs of students with dyslexia and only 31 per cent believed that remedial teachers were trained to teach students with dyslexia.

There is no doubt that provision for pupils with dyslexia is improving in Ireland. Strides have been made in public awareness, access to psychological assessment and availability of support from remedial and resource teachers. However, much remains to be done and for many students the support provided by the Dyslexia Association is still crucial.

DYSLEXIA ASSOCIATION OF IRELAND

Since its foundation in 1971, the Association has grown rapidly. It now has 39 branches, each of which runs extra-curricular reading classes and functions as a parent support group. Two full-time psychologists are employed at the national office in Suffolk Street, Dublin, where psycho-educational assessment is offered for children and adults. Group or individual tuition can be arranged for those who have been diagnosed with dyslexia in most areas of the country. Summer schools and special exam preparation classes are offered. A full-time course for adults with dyslexia is run in conjunction with FAS, the national training agency. This is the only course of its kind in Ireland and enables adults whose employment prospects have been hindered by dyslexia to acquire literacy and computer skills.

The Dyslexia Association has been providing in-service teacher training courses in the identification and treatment of dyslexia since 1979. This course has been updated and developed over the years and is taken by 400 teachers each year. New teaching programmes and approaches are evaluated and information is circulated frequently to both parents and teachers. The Association offers a tutorial service at a number of tertiary level institutions and a most heartening development is the increasing number of students with dyslexia successfully completing tertiary level courses.

The Association has spearheaded successful campaigns to have students with severe dyslexia made exempt from the study of Irish and continues to press for appropriate special arrangements for students in state exams.

Perhaps the most important function of the Association is that it provides a forum to express the needs of students and their parents, of adults with dyslexia, of concerned teachers at all levels and that it keeps the issue of dyslexia very much alive within the Irish education system.

ORGANIZATION

Dyslexia Association of Ireland
1 Suffolk Street
Dublin 2
Tel.: 353 1 6790276
Fax: 353 1 6790273
Email: info@dslexia.ie
Website: www.dyslexia.ie

CHAPTER AUTHOR

Anne Hughes
Dyslexia Association of Ireland
1 Suffolk Street
Dublin 2

DYSLEXIA IN ISRAEL

G. Malka Lipkin and Harry J. Lipkin

INTRODUCTION

Israel has free compulsory education with public schools available in both of Israel's official languages, Hebrew and Arabic. Nearly all children attend public schools in the language chosen by their parents. In Israel 8 per cent of the entire population of pupils are treated in the programme for treatment of children with special needs. This compares with 10 per cent in the USA and 14 per cent in Canada. The resources for pupils with learning disabilities are not separate, and those given specifically to dyslexic pupils cannot be identified.

In Israel one finds the same two approaches to dyslexia common elsewhere: (1) dyslexia is a learning disability which society must help children live with; and (2) dyslexia is a reading difficulty which can be overcome by proper teaching.

The Ministry of Education of Israel defines dyslexia as a disfunctioning from birth, that expresses itself in reading disability, which itself is a sub-category of a general heterogeneous group of learning disabilities, that includes attention problems, language disabilities, and mathematical capacity disability. The diagnosis is made within the educational system by psychologists, after early identification by the teacher. First grade teachers receive instruction from advisers and psychologists on identifying children with difficulty in reading, and how to help them to learn to read in an individual manner.

There is a support structure, of Matya teachers (acronym for Support Service Local and Regional), who receive instruction from professional advisers on helping the teachers cope with children having difficulty. In cases where this help is not sufficient and the gap increases between the pupil's mastery of reading in comparison with other pupils, the advisability of a psychological diagnosis is weighed.

In secondary school and in higher education, the process is similar, of identification of the disability and of adjusting teaching methods and examinations. In the examinations called 'Bagrut Tests' (matriculation examinations) there are certain dispensations for dyslexics according to the instructions of the psychologists, including having questions read aloud, a limited form of the tests, and extension of time for the test.

International Book of Dyslexia: A Guide to Practice and Resources. Edited by Ian Smythe, John Everatt and Robin Salter. ISBN 0-471-49646-4. © 2004 John Wiley & Sons, Ltd.

ISRAEL ORTON DYSLEXIA

An Israel Orton Dyslexia Society was founded in 1992 by a small group of volunteers, including Ms Bracha Weingrod. The present Director, David Finkelstein, joined the organization in 1994. Today there are almost 800 members. An active Centre runs a volunteer service that includes: an Open Ear, a library of articles, a listing of local professionals and organizations providing services for dyslexics and reprints of some of the materials from the International Dyslexia Society of the United States, of which the Israel Society is a member.

A modern approach (see, for example, the article by Joseph K. Torgesen, in *Perspectives*, International Dyslexia Association, Vol. 23, p. 27) focuses on methods to increase the word reading skills in dyslexic children through both preventive and remedial interventions. In Israel this approach is implemented by the first grade reading programme LITAF and the remedial reading programme TIKVA, which treat all children the same and provide adequate reading education for all. LITAF claims that all children can be taught to read in first and second grade and that there is no need to classify and segregate dyslexics at this stage.

Any attempt to delve further into the real situation of dyslexia in Israel leads to the same problems of reading education that have produced reading wars and myths everywhere. The use of myths about famous dyslexics to make children classified as dyslexic feel good about their reading problems has been questioned. For instance, no evidence supports the myth that Einstein was dyslexic. The modern approach used by LITAF in Israel attacks the reading problems directly, finds ways to solve them and enables the children to join the mainstream as normal children.

THE LITAF PROGRAMME

The LITAF system used in Israel may provide a unique contribution to our understanding of how to deal with the problem of dyslexia. This programme has a record of success over a 20-year period and is now in use in 300 schools in Israel, teaching 18,000 first grade pupils each year. There is no selection to remove children with learning disabilities from LITAF classes. LITAF succeeds in teaching all of them to read, including the dyslexics who are present in any normal population. This extensive reservoir of experience with real children in real classes deserves serious attention.

The LITAF programme for teaching reading, writing and comprehension, including grammatical structure, emphasizes the early identification of pupils having difficulties, analysis of the difficulties and of the specific weakness of each pupil, and their treatment. The source and particular name for the difficulties are not considered relevant.

The didactic and educational approach for a heterogeneous first grade class develops and strengthens the capacities needed to acquire reading with comprehension and writing. The pupil is spared the suffering commonly experienced by a pupil who finishes first grade without having mastered reading, e.g. the feeling that there are no answers, the frustration, the sorrow, the disgrace and the lowered self-esteem that cause suffering every day and every hour in school, in society, and even at home in the family. LITAF treats children with reading difficulties together with children who have already begun reading at age four and others at all levels in between, all in the same first grade class.

A new programme teaches both LITAF reading, writing, and reading comprehension for first grade, and also TIKVA (hope in Hebrew) remedial reading, reading comprehension and learning strategies for the same school for all grades in which LITAF had not been taught. All pupils of grades 2 to 6 needing remediation are identified; their teachers are then taught to teach their pupils to master reading at each grade level, with material adapted to that level. Teachers are taught and participate in intensive workshops, while their teachers model the work by working with the designated pupils so that the children in those schools will indeed NOT be left behind. This programme has recently been implemented in several schools.

The programme has been developed in Hebrew and in Arabic, and is now implemented in several schools. Plans to use the programme on a large scale for two major sections of the Israel Arab population were developed, but cancelled at the last minute due to bureaucratic problems at the Ministry of Education. There is hope that some form of the programme will be revived in the near future.

The work of LITAF is supported by the work of the major pioneers of understanding reading, Isabelle Liberman, Alvin Liberman, and Donald Shankweiler, as well as the work of other major contributors to understanding: Marilyn J. Adams, Keith Stanovich, David Share, Ram Frost, Susan Brady, Louisa Moats and Reid Lyon. TIKVA in its original form, in the seventh grade for students entering the junior high school system, and in its new form in the elementary school, is in line with the work of the above, plus that of Joseph Torgesen, Frank Vellutino and others.

ORGANIZATIONS

International Dyslexia Association (ORTON)
24A Alexander Hagadol
PO Box 6304
Hod Hasharon
Israel 45240
Tel.: +972 974 09646
Fax: +972 974 03160
Email: davidzvi@netvision.net.il
Website: www.orton-ida.org.il

CHAPTER AUTHORS

G. Malka Lipkin
University of Chicago
Chicago

Harry J. Lipkin
Professor of Physics
Weizmann Institute of Science
Rehovot, Israel
and
Israel Academy of Sciences and Humanities
Jerusalem
Israel

LITAF
Nira Altalef
Director
Education Services
Twin Tower 2
Jabotinsky 35
Ramat Gan
Israel 52511
Tel.: +972 3 7512370
Fax: +972 3 7512362
Email: litaf@zahav.net.il

DYSLEXIA IN ITALY

Giacomo Stella

INTRODUCTION

Developmental dyslexia has a recent history in Italy. Only 20 years ago it was very difficult to be recognized as dyslexic in regular schools as teachers did not receive any information on reading difficulties during their training. Children with reading difficulties were interpreted as lazy or having behavioural or emotional problems. In clinical settings it was rare to be assessed as dyslexic, as learning disabilities were attributed to psycho-emotional disturbances and the cognitive and neuropsychological approaches were not widely known. In the past two decades, research into this learning difficulty has grown rapidly both on the fundamental cognitive aspects involved in literacy acquisition and on its neuro-anatomical and neurophysiological basis.

In Italy, in the early 1980s the first research was published on the neuropsychological studies on dyslexia, but it was more than ten years before protocols were available for clinical evaluation. Until the 1990s children having difficulties in reading and spelling were not identified as dyslexic and received inappropriate remediation at school; if they did not have a language impairment history, remediation was in rehabilitation centres.

FEATURES OF ITALIAN ORTHOGRAPHY

Italian orthography is very regular. Most of the letters have a one-to-one correspondence with sounds and can be taught separately. There are sounds which have different representation depending on the phonological context and coded with multi-letters graphemes (such as K, or G) but rules are very stable. Italian orthography does not have homophones so during reading we do not encounter written words or morphemes that could be read in a different way. In our orthographic system, accent is the only phonetic feature not clearly represented. In most spoken Italian, word accent bears on the penultimate syllable, some-

International Book of Dyslexia: A Guide to Practice and Resources. Edited by Ian Smythe, John Everatt and Robin Salter. ISBN 0-471-49646-4. © 2004 John Wiley & Sons, Ltd.

times on the final one and sometimes on the first. The only occasion in which accent is orthographically represented is when it bears on the last syllable. During language acquisition Italian children can encounter some difficulty in reading aloud some words with the accent on the first syllable as they are trained to stress the non-accented words as the penultimate, e.g. *tavolo* ('table') that can be read as *tavòlo*, instead of *tàvolo*.

In spelling, the specificity of Italian is on the representation of so-called 'doubles' (standing for double letters such as in pizza or spaghetti). We use 'doubles' to represent the prolongation of the vowel and this is very important as this characteristic bears a distinctive phonetic trait.

Due to the regularity of the orthography, Italian children learn to read and spell very quickly. It may be for this reason that we find a lower incidence of dyslexia in the Italian population than in other countries. In the Italian literature we have different estimates ranging from 1.5 per cent to 5.5 per cent, depending on the testing material and the criteria used. Even if it is not easy to gain consensus on the incidence of dyslexia in our surveys, we estimate that 3.5 per cent of the school age population is dyslexic.

ASSESSMENT

Following Italian laws, a diagnosis can be made only by medical doctors and psychologists. No diagnosis can be certified by speech therapists or teachers.

Assessment includes psychological evaluation, language tests, reading and spelling tests, memory and attention tests, and arithmetic tests and has to be made in a clinical setting. A speech therapist usually participates in the assessment. Children are generally assessed in consultation with the family or with the teachers. In any case, schools are not allowed to refer children for assessment without the permission of the family.

The neuropsychological approach to evaluation is rapidly growing in Italy. Procedures for diagnosing children with learning difficulties are now taught to professionals at university in special training courses. Nevertheless, it is still very common to get a wrong diagnosis, due to the lack of knowledge among professionals and to the prevalence of the psycho-emotional approach to learning disabilities in general to developmental impairments.

TREATMENT AND REMEDIATION

Treatment has rules created by speech therapists, mostly working in the national health system. In general, they try to improve the phonological and meta-phonological processes. Computer-assisted therapy is used to help spelling and reading.

Specific remediation programmes given by school teachers do not exist and the school committee of the Associazione Italiana Dislessia (AID) is preparing some programmes to extend remediation to the schools and to ensure an adequate education for dyslexic children.

WHAT THE SCHOOLS ARE DOING

In Italy the school system is changing as we are moving from a centralized to a local organizational level. Until now, no official screening has been done by the government to identify learning difficulties, but now a number of schools are organizing early detection programmes themselves. The AID has made a huge contribution to the development of early detection and remediation programmes, but the possibility of detecting children at the early stages of literacy acquisition is still very low and is limited to some regions of the country in which the AID is well established. In Italy we do not have specific provision for dyslexic children. There is a general law for the integration of handicapped children in regular schools, and in some cases it can be used to obtain a special teacher for a few hours during the week (with a maximum of six hours per week).

Special teachers are not specifically trained for children with learning disabilities. They receive training to teach mentally retarded or sensory impaired children and they try to adapt their methods to the needs of dyslexic children, though in general the results are very poor.

Usually a special teacher trained for mental retardation adopts a total care attitude towards the child and tries to mediate the whole relationship: between regular teaching and knowledge acquisition. This is accepted at the very early stages after identification (in second grade), but can later be refused as the child experiences a feeling of inadequacy and of separation from classmates. Up to now, the school system has been very rigid and compensatory tools like computers, calculators, and other facilitators were not accepted in daily school work. They are admitted only during special training; the introduction of these aids in school activities is a major issue.

ADULT DYSLEXIA

Until now, very episodic experiences have been the case of adult dyslexics. We do not have any information on help for dyslexic Italian students, but maybe this is one of the reasons why in Italy this topic is underestimated and underdeveloped. The other reason certainly lies in the late development of the 'dyslexic movement' in Italy, as a number of adults are now calling the AID to ask for a re-assessment of their unsuccessful school career.

PARENTS

Some of the recent activities of the 'dyslexic movement' have produced negative effects with some parents, as up to now, they had been confused over the identification of their child's problem and on how to manage it. Since the AID was founded, the Social Problems committee has done a great deal to assist parents. The AID set up a help-line to give assistance to people, and calls were mostly from parents. At the time of writing, there are two established self-help programmes for parents.

THE DYSLEXIC MOVEMENT IN ITALY

The AID was founded in 1997 and since then a lot of initiatives have been carried out in order to raise awareness through the media. Conferences have taken place addressed to the general public, TV appearances have been made, seminars have been held in many schools, and intensive courses for teachers and professionals have been introduced.

Our association, in order to respond quickly and efficiently to the different issues, is divided into three committees: Social Problems (mostly parents and adult dyslexics), School (teachers), and Professionals (speech therapists, psychologists, child psychiatrists, and neurologists). Each committee undertakes specific issues such as demanding school provision acts, protocols for assessment and self-help programmes.

Up to now, the AID has around 1,000 members from 16 different provincial areas, covering 12 of the 20 regions.

ORGANIZATIONS

Associazione Italia Dislessia
Via Testoni 1
40123 Bologne
Italy
Tel./Fax: +39 51 270 578/+39 51 274 784
Email: AID@dislessia.it
Website: www.dislessia.it

Laboratorio di Neuropsicologia
Unita di Neurologia
Arcispedale S. Maria Nuova
Reggio Emilia
Italy
Tel.: +39 522 296 031

Centro Reperto Internazionale Demenze
Reggio Emilia
Albinea
Italy
Tel: +39 522 348 845
Email: enrico.ghidoni@carpi.nettuno.it

CHAPTER AUTHOR

Giacomo Stella
Associazione Italiana Dislessia
Via Testoni 1
40123 Bologne
Italy
Email: AID@dislessia.it

DYSLEXIA IN JAPAN

Eiko Todo

JAPAN: CONTEXT

In Japan dyslexia is considered as one of the symptoms of LD (learning disabilities). It was not until 10 years ago that the true movement towards recognition of LD started under the leadership of Professor Kazuhiko Ueno. Parents groups were formed to gather information and to investigate the possibilities. The notion of LD is still confused although the Ministry of Health and Welfare and Ministry of Education have come up with the definition, respectively, in 1997 and 1999. Many other symptoms such as ADHD, autism, and mental retardation are still included at the level of LD Gakkai (Academic Circle) or Parents Association. Incidence of dyslexia is considered to be relatively low compared to English-speaking countries (3–4 per cent in Japan against 10–12 per cent in the UK). This is not a concrete figure as there is no standardized criterion for assessment of dyslexia in Japan nor a dedicated assessment to undertake the survey.

Lack of information and knowledge, the clear structure of the Japanese language where there are only five vowels and one *kana* per syllable and the existence of *kanji* characters which express the meaning, all these combine together and contribute to lowering the percentage of incidence of dyslexia in Japan.

LEGISLATION AND POLICIES

There is currently no legislation concerning dyslexia or LD in Japan. But there are positive moves to start a programme of special educational needs (SEN) within the framework of regular classes. Unfortunately the main focus is on the physically disabled, the blind and the partially sighted, the deaf and hard of hearing and on the mentally retarded and so forth, and neither LD nor dyslexia is mentioned. This is intended only for the elementary school and lower secondary school (i.e. up to age 15). In 2001, a budget was allotted to

International Book of Dyslexia: A Guide to Practice and Resources. Edited by Ian Smythe, John Everatt and Robin Salter. ISBN 0-471-49646-4. © 2004 John Wiley & Sons, Ltd.

the research into LD in all 47 prefectures in Japan. The purpose of the research is to designate a school per prefecture and investigate the number of LD in each school and then to look for a teaching method.

DEFINITION AND TERMINOLOGY

The word 'dyslexia' in Japan is purely used for adult alexia as a medical term. In educational terms, LD is widely used in Japan. The definition for LD in Japan is laid down by the Ministry of Education and Ministry of Health and Welfare, and includes dyslexia, dysgraphia, dyscalculia and dyspraxia. We try to use the term developmental dyslexia in order to differentiate from dyslexia which is caused by accident or illness and LD which in Japan sometimes includes retardation, autism, ADHD and epilepsy.

IDENTIFICATION AND ASSESSMENT

Most local educational authorities rely only on psychological tests such as WISC-III to measure the difference between verbal IQ and performance IQ. Specialist tests include WISC-III, diagram tracing of Gesell, anomia, vocabulary test and phonetic recognition by speech therapist and clinical diagnosis such as handwriting, and language comprehension. It is similar to the Bangor test in the UK. In short, there is not yet a standardized assessment for dyslexia in Japan.

INTERVENTION AND RESOURCES

For children with special educational needs there are classes outside ordinary classes for the speech impaired and emotionally disturbed. These children commute to these classes once a week. Some LD children are included. The class for the emotionally disturbed was designed to deal with children with autism (Asperger) and ADHD in order to train them in social skills in groups of three or four children. There are some dyslexic children in speech-impaired classes but they are usually not taught correctly unless the teacher in charge is experienced.

TEACHER TRAINING

Teachers from ordinary classes are assigned to these SEN classes for one day. They have a brief training on how to operate the hearing aid and to undertake some hearing tests. The new teachers have a training session for SEN before joining the schools in the form of a lecture.

ADVOCACY GROUPS

Advocacy groups in Japan are the LD Gakkai (Academic Circle) and the Parents Association.

EXAMS AND CURRICULUM PROVISIONS

There are no provisions for assistance in exams. There are some cases where private high schools allow students to take an oral exam but actually none of the dyslexic students were allowed in to these schools.

THE WAY AHEAD

NPO EDGE (the Japan Dyslexia Society) has been approved to undertake various support tasks for dyslexic children and adults. The aim of the NPO is to facilitate the lives of dyslexic people and their priority is to prepare a system which is affordable and manageable. The first thing the NPO has to cope with is to prepare a check list, a screening test and an assessment test, followed by educational materials and knowledge for teachers and parents to use at school and home. The next step would be to consider English teaching methods for children who have been diagnosed at junior high school. Then to prepare the provision for the exams, work with private schools to include dyslexic children in their schools, and prepare a working environment for dyslexic people.

Collaboration between the parties involved is another area to be explored. Education, health and welfare, employment and other administrative bodies should all get together to work out a practical system for dyslexic people. Diet (the Japanese parliament) members are forming a parliamentary group across all the parties to discuss policies concerning SEN and dyslexia.

Media coverage of dyslexia is increasing. A famous actress who is proven to be very clever has written in her new publication that she has dyscalculia. This is the first time in Japan someone famous has admitted having an LD.

REFERENCE

Ministry of Education (2001) *To Encourage Zest for Living: Special Education in Japan*. Tokyo: Ministry of Education.

ORGANIZATIONS

NPO EDGE Japan Dyslexia Society
Minato NPO House
4-7-14
Roppongi
Minato-ku
Tokyo
Japan 106-0032
Email: info@npo-edge.jp

Dr Junko Kato
LD Gakkai
Dyslexia Section
Clinic Kato
Japan

Masayoshi Tsuge
Senior Specialist
Special Support Education Division
Ministry of Education
Tokyo
Japan

CHAPTER AUTHOR

Eiko Todo
NPO EDGE – Japan Dyslexia Society
2-31-7-1002
Jingumae
Shibuya-ku
Tokyo
Japan 150-0001
Email: todo@todoplan.co.jp

DYSLEXIA IN JORDAN

Radi Waqfi

INTRODUCTION

The interest in dealing with learning difficulties/disabilities (LDs) in Jordan stemmed from the initiative of HRH Princess Sarvath who chairs the Board of Trustees of the Princess Sarvath College in Amman. In December 1992, the College concluded an agreement with the Canadian authorities to train a number of teachers in the field of LD in Canada and in Jordan over three years. The ultimate goal of this project is to offer remedial services to the great number of our students who suffer from LD without receiving any proper attention. In 1994, the College signed an agreement with the Ministry of Education in Jordan to train a number of its teachers in this field. In 1995 the National Centre for Learning Difficulties (NCLD) was established on the premises of the College.

Training the teachers in the field of learning difficulties is compatible with the recommendations of the National Conference for the Development of Education (1987) in Jordan, which emphasized the improvement of the quality of education. Democratic education, which caters for the needs and abilities of children and solves their problems, is a priority in this project. Suffering from LD will adversely affect the learning process and consequently lead to under-achievement and drop-out if not remedied.

SCHOOLS AND LANGUAGES

According to the *Statistical Year Book* of the Ministry of Education (2000), there are 4,804 schools in Jordan under the control of four different authorities: Ministry of Education (2,833), private sector (1,733), UNRWA (192) and other governmental authorities (46). The Ministry of Education, by law, has been mandated to provide curricula and technical supervision. The total number of students is 1,387,300 which is almost one-third of the total population, taught by 67,696 teachers. Around 51 per cent of the students are boys and 49 per cent are girls. Some of these schools are co-educational schools, while others

International Book of Dyslexia: A Guide to Practice and Resources. Edited by Ian Smythe, John Everatt and Robin Salter. ISBN 0-471-49646-4. © 2004 John Wiley & Sons, Ltd.

are segregated schools, especially for the 13–18 year age group. Basic and compulsory education consists of the first 10 years while the secondary stage consists of two more years. After that, the students sit a general examination held by the Ministry of Education. Those who attain high averages can pursue university studies.

Arabic, which is an alphabetic language, is the official language in Jordan and it is the medium of instruction. English is taught as a second language from the fifth elementary grade. Teaching English beginning in the first year at school is a new educational policy adopted by the Ministry of Education two years ago and is gradually being implemented.

LEGISLATION AND POLICY

Public laws, especially the Education Act No. 3 of 1994 implemented by the Ministry of Education, and the Protection of the Handicapped Act (PHA) No. 12 of 1993, implemented by the Ministry of Social Welfare, protect the legal rights of students suffering from handicapping conditions to equal opportunities to receive the appropriate education in the public schools. No special regulations concerning LD are mentioned in any of these laws. The Ministry of Education and the Ministry of Health are mandated to assess and diagnose disabilities in general. Public schools and higher education institutions are required to prepare appropriate conditions necessary to facilitate the education of the disabled. However, students with LD, like other disabled students, have the right to be placed in regular classrooms as long as their disabilities are compatible with this setting. Otherwise, they are taught in resource rooms or special classes depending on the severity of their disability.

DEFINITION AND TERMINOLOGY

'Learning disabilities' is the generic or umbrella term used to cover a heterogeneous group of disorders related to a certain category of special education. 'Learning difficulties' as a term is preferred to other terms such as dyslexia or learning disabilities because (1) 'dyslexia' which originally means severe reading difficulties was coined and primarily used by neurological and medical professions focusing on genetics, brain damage and minimal brain dysfunction. Teachers who do the assessment, diagnosis and intervention do not know unfamiliar and what may be vague medical terms; and (2) 'disabilities', when translated literally into Arabic, means handicaps, which is not acceptable and frightening to the student and his or her family. Thus, 'disabilities' is translated into an Arabic word which means difficulties when translated into English. These terms, such as mild, moderate or severe learning difficulties in reading and/or writing, are the prevailing terms used in Jordan. As an alternative to dyslexia some use specific learning difficulty and others use severe reading difficulty.

Severe learning difficulty in reading, as understood at the National Centre for Learning Difficulties, is a persistent difficulty in learning the components of written words and sentences. It is of constitutional origin, presumed to be a central nervous system dysfunction and not due to intellectual inadequacy or to lack of proper cultural, emotional or pedagogical conditions. It is cognitive in nature, manifested in the form of visual-to-verbal coding, spatial directional confusion, short-term memory and sequential ordering affecting written language skills, namely reading, spelling and handwriting. Although this difficulty might occur concomitantly with other handicapping factors whether physical, social, emotional or educational, it is not the direct result of these factors. These difficulties are developmental disorders and are more common among boys.

A student with severe learning difficulty in reading might show unusual symptoms concerning reading habits: tension movements, losing his place, holding material close, insecurity, word recognition errors, omissions, additions, reversals or substitutions of words and letters, mispronunciations, transpositions and weak comprehension. In addition, reading is characterized by a high-pitched voice, ignored or misinterpreted punctuation and word-by-word reading.

IDENTIFICATION AND ASSESSMENT

The NCLD from its inception aimed to take on the responsibility of promoting public awareness about LD, to function as a national diagnostic referral centre for children referred by families or schools and to be a training centre for teachers who wish to become resource teachers at their schools.

Ten years ago the Ministry of Education began, at a limited number of basic education schools, the policy of 'resource rooms' in order to provide supportive teaching to underachievers regardless of the labelling of those students. It was the beginning of the adoption of special education principles and methods.

The real start in handling the problem of learning difficulties began in 1996 with the first group of resource teachers who graduated from the NCLD, where they were trained to administer a battery of tests either adapted or developed and standardized by Jordanian scholars to fit the Jordanian context. This battery consists of formal tests and informal inventories.

Formal tests used in Jordan:

- the Wechsler Intelligence Scale for Children (WISC-III) under licence from The Psychological Corporation;
- a perceptual group of tests (norm-referenced) which assess and diagnose any of the following: perceptual discrimination, auditory analysis skills, visual analysis, sequential auditory memory, auditory memory span and visual motor integration;
- the Diagnosis Test of Basic Arabic skills (criterion-referenced);
- the Diagnosis Test of Basic Mathematics skills (criterion-referenced).

Informal inventories used are:

- classroom readings inventory;
- informal reading analysis inventory;
- checklist of learning difficulties symptoms.

Resource teachers are encouraged to use the checklist in screening new students and identifying those at risk. Pre-referral interventions are suggested by a planning team at the school to the classroom teacher, to ensure that the student has been appropriately taught in his classroom setting. If the strategies provided are not helpful, the student will be referred for assessment. Resource teachers, psychology counsellors, Arabic teachers and classroom teachers participate in this process. The permission of the family and at least some family participation are necessary. The assessment process should be comprehensive and should take into account different criteria for determining that the student suffers from LD such as a significant discrepancy between expected and actual achievement in one or more of the following: basic oral and silent reading skills, listening comprehension, reading comprehension, mathematics and style of learning (auditory, visual or motor). The team also takes into account that those difficulties are not a result of mental defects, visual, hearing or motor defects or behavioural, educational or socio-economic factors.

Jordan's educational system is still far from generalizing this procedure. The procedure is still limited to those schools which have resource teachers. Two local studies were conducted in Jordan. Learning difficulties, according to these studies, are estimated to account for around 7.5 per cent of the students.

INTERVENTION AND RESOURCES

Assessment, as a necessary prerequisite to good teaching, without remediation is a waste of time, if not harmful to the student. Its importance stems from providing a data baseline or a starting point for intervention. If the student was diagnosed by observations, meetings, tests and achievement records to be reading disabled (dyslexic), the same team (which might include other necessary personnel) start preparing the individual education plan (IEP). This plan should address his or her needs (weaknesses) and bolster his or her strengths. The IEP should determine what to teach and how to teach on a daily basis and in accordance with long-term and short-term behavioural instructional objectives. The IEP in its initial form should be considered a tentative one. Interactive assessment and diagnostic teaching are good methods to determine the adequacy of the initial form of the IEP or whether there is a need to adapt it.

The least restrictive environment for the student's replacement should be decided. The severity of the problem determines replacement; if it is mild, the student receives intervention in his or her classroom, if it is moderate or severe, he or she attends a resource room or special classroom either part or most of the time. Private centres working in the field of assessment and intervention of students with LD are beginning to emerge, though not on a large scale.

TEACHER TRAINING

Training is implemented in two forms: the first is a general course where training aims at enhancing the awareness of parents, teachers, supervisors and administrators regarding the problem of learning difficulties. Several two-day and four-day workshops were carried out for different audiences to explain the concept of LD.

The second kind of training is a specialization core where training aims at preparing specialists in the field of learning difficulties, especially for those who aspire to become resource room teachers. Participants receive intensive theoretical and practical training for a whole scholastic year. This training includes required theoretical courses amounting to 21 credit hours (CH), practical training for six CH, and elective courses for six CH. Teachers who are admitted to this course are BA degree holders in psychology or education. Those who hold a BA degree in other fields are required to study three prerequisite courses of nine CH in education and psychology. A higher diploma in learning difficulties is granted to successful graduates. Special consideration is paid to the practical side. Students are required to administer the battery of tests and prepare a field case study as a graduation project.

In addition to the NCLD, three Jordanian universities have special education departments where graduates and post-graduate studies are delivered.

ADVOCACY GROUPS

The NCLD started functioning on an awareness level. A series of talks and meetings on different media and in workshops were undertaken. The only formal advocacy group existing in Jordan is the Arab Association for Learning Difficulties (AALD). This Association was formed through the Regional Seminar that was held on an initiative from the NCLD in co-operation with the Ministry of Education. Delegates from 13 Arab countries attended that seminar. The AALD took its formal form in December 2000, and it is now licensed to issue a half-yearly journal specializing in the field of LD. Membership of the AALD is open to all concerned individuals from all the Arab countries. It is hoped that AALD efforts, together with NCLD efforts, will form an active agency to protect the rights of students with LD and to enable them to pursue their academic studies in an educational medium that caters for their needs and abilities.

THE WAY AHEAD

Learning difficulties including dyslexia are still not handled properly in the Arab region. The NCLD is the only centre of its kind; it is our vision that the NCLD becomes a regional centre serving the Arab region, especially in training resource teachers.

ORGANIZATION

National Centre for Learning Difficulties (NCLD)
Princess Sarvath College
PO Box 926380
Amman 11190
Jordan
Tel./fax: 962 6 5151293
Email: Dean@sarvath.index.edu.jo

CHAPTER AUTHOR

Radi Waqfi
Dean
Princess Sarvath College
PO Box 926380
Amman 11190
Jordan
Tel./fax: 962 6 5151293
Email: Dean@sarvath.index.edu.jo

DYSLEXIA IN KENYA

William Eric Ferguson

INTRODUCTION

Kenya is a vast country where schools are in the cities and isolated far out in the countryside. The school system has two sectors: these are state-run schools and an independent sector. I work within the independent sector so it is this aspect of Kenyan education that I know most about. Most of the independent schools have a learning support department. There are schools run by the state for children who have recognizable physical disabilities. Many are English-medium schools. In these establishments all subject teaching, apart from foreign languages, is in English.

It seems that for the present the dyslexic may best be served by the independent sector. This is because many of the schools follow the British National Curriculum or that of the USA or other European countries. Another reason is that of providing for need.

Dyslexic children, despite living in isolated parts of the country and being in Africa can still have the educational opportunity to develop their potential. Many of the schools are 'dyslexic-friendly'. Here the curriculum has been adapted to the needs of the dyslexic who can have their difficulties targeted as well as follow mainstream courses and sit the same examinations as their non-dyslexic peers. The teachers thus employed have often been able to work with colleagues to develop educational opportunities for the dyslexic.

DEFINITIONS AND INCIDENCE

The definition Kenya uses to classify children as being dyslexic is that given by the British Dyslexia Association (BDA). The prevalence is about 10 per cent of children and, according to an in-school study, more boys are dyslexic than girls.

At primary level much work is done in giving these children help in class, as well as individual support and differential work practices to take them forward. There are schools which allow the dyslexic to take computers or word processors into the classroom. These

International Book of Dyslexia: A Guide to Practice and Resources. Edited by Ian Smythe, John Everatt and Robin Salter. ISBN 0-471-49646-4. © 2004 John Wiley & Sons, Ltd.

schools offer typing courses to develop word processing skills. Teachers have found that the dyslexic's typing speed is much quicker than their handwritten note-taking. Teachers believe this is good motivation and they have seen the dyslexic student achieving better marks and grades than previously. A similar pattern of teaching takes place in senior schools. Dyslexic students taking IGCSE have applied and succeeded in being granted extra time by the British examining boards.

ASSESSMENT

The Specific Learning Difficulties (SpLD) teachers in some schools do the initial assessment. They are likely to use the Aston Index and other teacher-based assessments. The policy of other schools is to refer the child directly to an educational psychologist for assessment. Should a pupil require a speech therapist, then this service is available in Nairobi.

Teachers are continually upgrading their skills. This is done through curriculum development meetings held annually for teachers. Some teachers are following distance-learning courses for the Hornsby diploma or at the Master's degree level. The main problem seems to be a feeling of isolation from the providers. Several teachers have formed a group to give support to each other. Many teachers are members of the BDA or the International Dyslexia Association (IDA). In November 2001 teachers from all over Kenya attended a one-day dyslexic conference.

Parents were asked to input their ideas and it was surprising to find that some of them felt that schools were not fully aware of all the aspects of being dyslexic. Parents are not as able to help their children because they do not know where to find help and advice. Obtaining books is not easy in Nairobi and a lot of searching was needed to find very useful books. Many parents did not know that books about dyslexia were available in Kenya.

THE WAY AHEAD

Some parents felt that a dyslexic centre composed of trained teachers from different schools and parents would bring together excellence to focus on providing help and information. This body could hold an annual meeting, have a website and use email to have open discussion and keep everyone informed. To this end a website has been created: www.weferdyslexia.8m.net.

At present there are no facilities for dyslexic adults in Kenya. Kenya has begun to build a firm foundation for giving help to the dyslexic, but there is much still to be done. Parents and teachers working together is an issue that is likely to benefit the dyslexic in Kenya.

CONTACTS

William Ferguson
Email: wefer1999@yahoo.com

Parent contact: Annete Lanjouw
Email: Alanjouw@awfle.org

CHAPTER AUTHOR

William Ferguson
8 Braeburn Court
Leigh
Lancashire WN7 5BE
Email: wefer1999@yahoo.com

DYSLEXIA IN LUXEMBOURG

Lucien Bertrand

INTRODUCTION

The remedial teaching of dyslexic children in Luxembourg has, for a good many years, been mainly in the hands of teachers who have been specifically trained to offer support to children with learning difficulties. The training takes different forms and lasts for different periods, varying between several years and several months. At present a large number of specialist teachers of dyslexic children are to be found within the Service Ré-Educatif Ambulatoire (SREA) (a peripatetic remedial teaching service), which was created in 1993 within the framework of L'Education Différenciée (a special school system established under the Ministry of Education). In addition to providing assistance in the classroom for children with specific needs who are integrated into mainstream education, the service ensures that dyslexic children receive support. Such support may be offered in the schools themselves or in the offices of the service outside school hours. Support follows the principles of differentiation and meets the specific individual needs of the child. In line with the current philosophy of educational integration, such children continue with normal schooling. If necessary, other professionals such as psychometricians, psychologists, speech therapists, etc., join the remedial teachers involved, so that at present children who need it can be guaranteed the support of a team.

THE LUXEMBOURG SCHOOL SYSTEM

In this context, it should be noted that the Luxembourg school system has particular constraints for young children. Half the children in primary education have a mother tongue other than Luxemburgish. Reading and writing are taught in German and during the second year of primary school, students begin to learn French. This means that a good many chil-

International Book of Dyslexia: A Guide to Practice and Resources. Edited by Ian Smythe, John Everatt and Robin Salter. ISBN 0-471-49646-4. © 2004 John Wiley & Sons, Ltd.

dren have difficulties at school without being in any way dyslexic. In our view, not all the children for whom the learning of languages presents difficulties are dyslexic. In order to talk about dyslexia, learning difficulties in relation to reading and writing must occur within the child together with problems of visual and auditory perception, difficulties at the level of spatio-temporal organization, laterality or self-confidence.

DEFINITION

Let us recall here the definition of dyslexia as we understand it: we talk about dyslexia from the moment when, under normal school conditions and despite the best efforts of the adults working with him, a child of normal intelligence either does not succeed in learning to read and write or makes insignificant progress in that area. Generally speaking, at the same time the same child shows no particular difficulties in other subjects. Without going into detail here as to the possible causes of such a problem, it must be emphasized that multiple cause theories are always to be preferred to single cause theories.

Any intervention will therefore be preceded by a searching diagnosis covering different aspects: the child's medical and developmental history, intelligence level, skill at visual and auditory differentiation, test of laterality, evaluation of the level of spatio-temporal development, examination of emotional development and his or her relationships with others.

SUPPORT PROGRAMMES

Any support programme takes account of the problems found by the diagnostic tests. In addition to offering an appropriate remedial programme the child must be given global support and any specific needs must be taken into account. It goes without saying that for such children, who are deeply frustrated and hurt in themselves, expectations of achievement and performance are very greatly reduced and we need to create a situation in which they can learn successfully and rediscover in themselves the motivation needed for a fresh effort.

The remedial teacher will not be the one to correct the spelling mistakes; rather he or she will be the catalyst of action by the teacher in class. Within the framework thus described the child in difficulty must be given the opportunity of improving his or her self-image, his or her physical and psychological balance, his or her orientation in space and time and his or her visual, auditory and tactile perception. Rhythmic exercises as well as dance and mime will be useful to complete the work, which is based on the child and not on school programmes. Any working period will finish with relaxation exercises and a verbal account of what has taken place.

The attitude of the remedial teacher, therefore, will above all be that of a helper, friend and confidant. The remedial teacher will know that it is not by setting even more exercises that he or she can help a child in difficulty but by his or her own commitment and real investment in the critical school situation in which the child is placed. It is from the remedial teacher that the child will be able to draw the support necessary to achieve success.

DYSPEL ASBL.

In addition to the formal structure of help, a local support group can be a useful resource for parents and teachers for information or to discuss concerns and frustrations. Dyspel asbl., the dyslexia and special needs group in Luxembourg, aims to raise awareness of these children who require a different style of teaching, to provide information and to support parents as they try to find the best educational solution for their child. It has a library of resource material and can network and liaise with professionals and schools.

As well as holding talks and support meetings, Dyspel has produced a multilingual book for parents and teachers entitled *Dyslexia: Strategies for Success in School* in French, German and English. This provides information on diagnosis and how to help children to learn better in the classroom. Also, Dyspel is running a part-time post-graduate certificate course for teachers of multilingual children, which will give classroom teachers and other professionals the skills required to help children with specific learning difficulties achieve their potential.

ORGANIZATION

Dyspel asbl.
12, am Daerchen
L-5336 Moutfort
Luxembourg
Email: mccarth@pt.lu

CHAPTER AUTHOR

Lucien Bertrand
Service Ré-Educatif Ambulatoire
9 rue Federspiel
L-1512 Luxembourg

DYSLEXIA IN MALAYSIA

Caroline Gomez

INTRODUCTION

Malaysia is a relatively young nation, having gained independence from the British in 1957. It is a multi-ethnic society with a population of 23 million people. The Malays form the majority group (13.5 million). This is followed by the Chinese (5.6 million), Indians (1.6 million) and others (0.75 million) (*Malaysia Yearbook of Statistics*, 2000). About one-fifth of the Malaysian population are children: 2,931,847 attend primary schools while 1,999,371 are studying in secondary schools.

Education plays a vital role in achieving the country's vision of developing the full potential of the individual and fulfilling the aspiration of the Malaysian nation. Compulsory education is implemented from the ages of 6 to 17. The 1996 Education Act ensures the access to pre-school education of all children between the ages of 5 and 6. The primary school level covers a period of six years from Standard 1 to Standard 6. This is followed by three years of lower secondary school (Form 1–Form 3) and two years of upper secondary school (Form 4–Form 5). At the end of Form 5, students sit their O levels, after which students can choose to take their education to the post-secondary level which comprises another two years of formal education (Lower 6 and Upper 6). Having completed their A levels in Upper 6, students can apply for tertiary education at colleges and universities based on the criteria determined by the Education Ministry.

LANGUAGES

The national language is Bahasa Malaysia (BM). Bahasa Malaysia is also the home language of the majority group – the Malays. Most Malaysian Chinese speak Mandarin, or several other Chinese dialects such as Cantonese, Hokkien, Hakka, Teo Chew, and Hainanese. The majority of Malaysian Indians speak either Tamil or other Indian dialects,

International Book of Dyslexia: A Guide to Practice and Resources. Edited by Ian Smythe, John Everatt and Robin Salter. ISBN 0-471-49646-4. © 2004 John Wiley & Sons, Ltd.

for example, Malayalem, Hindi, Punjabi, and Telegu. Generally, Malaysians are trilinguals or bilinguals at the very least. The medium of instruction in national schools[1] is the Malay language (BM). However, in the national-type schools where Chinese and Tamil serve as the medium of instruction,[2] Bahasa Malaysia is taught as a compulsory subject. English is the second official language in Malaysia. Therefore, it is taught in all schools as a compulsory second language.

LEGISLATION AND POLICIES

The National Philosophy of Education (1989) states that 'education in Malaysia is an ongoing effort towards further developing the potential of individuals in a holistic and integrated manner so as to produce individuals who are intellectually, spiritually, emotionally, and physically balanced' (p. 5). Malaysia's education system is embodied in the national ideology or the Rukunegara. The underlying objectives of the Rukunegara are to do the following:

• to develop a united nation within a plural society;
• to develop a democratic society through a constitutionally elected Parliament;
• to develop a just society with equal opportunities for all;
• to develop a progressive society orientated towards science and modern technology.

Education in Malaysia is governed by five acts, one of which is the Education Act 1996 which replaces the former 1961 Education Act (*Malaysia Education Guide*, 2000). The new Education Act 1996 is a major educational reform undertaken by the Malaysian government to provide a high standard of education to all communities in the country. This includes children with special educational needs. Prior to the 1996 Act, the special needs of blind, deaf and physically handicapped children were being met. However, the needs of children with less obvious special needs were being neglected.

In the beginning of 2001, a working panel was set up to initiate the National Dyslexia Programme in Malaysia. This comprises ministry officials from the Department of Special Needs Education, dyslexia specialists from the Universiti Putra Malaysia, clinical psychologists, pediatricians, SEN teachers, speech therapists and parents. Apart from the educational, medical and lay teams collaborating for the advancement of dyslexia awareness in Malaysia, legal parties also corroborate this work. The Malaysian Bar Council is working on a memorandum on legislation for the education of individuals with disabilities. This memorandum encompasses the needs and rights of children with specific learning difficulties.

DEFINITION

The concept of specific developmental dyslexia is very much in its infancy in Malaysia, albeit it is fast gaining public attention. Here the term has not yet been churned in the lexical oven and as such lacks sophistication and complexity. The general public seems to use the term 'dyslexia' in a broad and simple sense to mean children who are 'stuck with print'. The local usage of the term tends to coincide with the definition of the World Federation of Neurology (1968) which asserts that dyslexia is 'a disorder in children who, despite conventional classroom experience, fail to attain the language skills of reading, writing, and spelling commensurate with their intellectual abilities'.

The Ministry of Education prefers the term 'specific learning difficulties' as it is a more functional definition. Their view of children with specific learning difficulties is in line with the United Kingdom's Special Needs Code of Practice (DFE, 1994) definition which refers to children who have significant difficulties in reading, writing, spelling or manipulating numbers, which are not typical of their general level of performance. They may gain some skills in some subjects quickly and demonstrate a high level of ability orally, yet may encounter sustained difficulty in gaining literacy or numeracy skills. Such children can become severely frustrated and may also have emotional and/or behavioural difficulties.

TERMINOLOGY

The panel responsible for the National Dyslexia programme has come up with its own abridged description of specific learning difficulties or 'disleksia' as it is known in Bahasa Malaysia. Tentatively, the operational definition of 'disleksia' refers to children who have a general level of performance which is similar to or above other children but have significant difficulty in fluent and accurate word reading and spelling.

PREVALENCE

To date, no research evidence is available on the prevalence of dyslexia in Malaysia. A pilot study (Gomez, 2000) conducted in a representative primary school of 2,000 pupils near Kuala Lumpur indicated that 7 per cent of Standard 2 Malay pupils had marked phonological reading difficulties (dyslexia). Although this study is an isolated case, it reveals that there are children with specific reading difficulties (dyslexia) in Malaysia. Many Malaysian parents are becoming more aware of dyslexia and suspect their children are dyslexic. They are continually seeking help from the Education Ministry and professionals in this field. Their cries for help and dialogues with top ministry officials from the Department of Special Needs Education have led to the initiation of a dyslexia programme at the national level.

IDENTIFICATION AND ASSESSMENT

Identification in primary schools

Presently there are no Malaysian standardized instruments to identify children with specific reading difficulties. In March 2001, the Ministry of Education officials from the Department of Special Needs collaborated with professionals from the Universiti Putra Malaysia (UPM) to formulate a checklist for screening all Malaysian children in Standard 1 for specific reading difficulties (dyslexia). The checklist (known as 'Senarai Semak Disleksia') consists of three elements: (i) pupils' level of mastery in reading and writing (spelling) and numeracy skills (difficulties); (ii) teachers'/parents' perception of pupils' abilities (strengths); and (iii) predictors of dyslexia. The 'Senarai Semak Disleksia' is issued to both the class teacher and parents of Standard 1 children. This screening instrument is currently being piloted in several primary schools nationwide.

Assessment in primary and secondary schools

Similar to identification, assessment of children with specific learning difficulties ('disleksia') in primary and secondary schools is not available. No Malaysian standardized assessment is yet available. The panel of experts of the National Dyslexia Programme are presently formulating a Dyslexia Reading Test to assess children who have been screened. This assessment instrument is still in its early days of development.

INTERVENTION AND RESOURCES

Thus far, interventions and resources for Malaysian children with dyslexia are limited. Although many enthusiastic parents, Rotary Clubs and NGOs have been supportive of the needs of children with dyslexia, the help rendered is rather basic and small-scale. Only recently the Education Ministry, after being spurred on by the demands of parents and informed others, has embarked on a National Dyslexia Programme. Hopefully, with the keen involvement of the Malaysian government, greater intervention measures will be developed and greater resources will be made available to the masses of children with dyslexia.

TEACHER TRAINING

There is acute need for all Malaysian teachers to be made aware of specific learning difficulties if help is to be made available for children with dyslexia in mainstream schools. Teachers need training in the appropriate knowledge and skills to facilitate identification and intervention. The Specialist Teacher Training College in Kuala Lumpur has long-term and short-term courses to train teachers in Special Educational Needs, inclusive of dyslexia. A few local universities are initiating courses in dyslexia to increase awareness and train teachers in this specialized area.

ADVOCACY GROUPS

Parent support groups and NGOs have been instrumental in advancing dyslexia awareness in Malaysia. The Kuala Lumpur Dyslexia Association is a charitable organization concerned with the education and welfare of dyslexic children and adults. Since its inception in 1995, the association has been responsible for conducting seminars and workshops to educate the community about dyslexia and other specific learning difficulties. The centre also conducts psychological and educational assessments to diagnose children with dyslexia. Once their dyslexia has been verified by a clinical psychologist, these children are offered tutoring in Bahasa Malaysia, English and Mathematics. The tuition is conducted individually or in small groups by skilled teachers trained in multi-sensory methods. The Bureau of Learning Difficulties (BOLD) in Penang provides similar facilities for dyslexics.

THE WAY AHEAD

With the Malaysian government taking a positive and strong lead, nationwide help for children with dyslexia is underway. However, screening and assessment instruments together with intervention procedures take a while to be implemented. So far, help for children with dyslexia has been scarce and isolated. Those living in Kuala Lumpur and Penang have benefited from the initiatives of proactive parents and NGOs. In the near future the Malaysian government, collaborating with universities, teacher training colleges, NGOs, psychologists, medical experts, speech therapists, researchers and parents, will further propel dyslexia awareness, identification, and remediation to the foreground.

NOTES

1 This is a government or government-aided school using the national language as the main medium of instruction and English is a compulsory subject of instruction. The teaching of Chinese or Tamil is made available if there is a request from at least 15 parents of the pupils in the school.
2 This is a government or government-aided school using Chinese or Tamil as the main medium of instruction and both the national and English languages are compulsory subjects of instruction.

REFERENCES

DFE (1994) *The Code of Practice for the Identification and Assessment of Special Educational Needs*. London: DFE Publication Centre.
Gomez, C.A. (2000) Identifying phonologically-based reading difficulties (dyslexia) in Malaysia children learning to read in English. Unpublished PhD thesis, University of Manchester.
Malaysia Education Guide (2000) 4th edition. Kuala Lumpur: Challenger Concept Publishers.
Malaysia Year Book of Statistics (2000) Kuala Lumpur: Department of Statistics.
World Federation of Neurology (1968) *Report of Research Group on Dyslexia and the World Illiteracy*. Dallas: WFN.

ORGANIZATIONS

Dr Haniz Bin Ibrahim
Assistant Director
Planning and Research Division
Tkt. 3 Blok G Selatan
Pusat Bandar Damansara
50 604 Kuala Lumpur
Malaysia
Tel.: (603) 2583704

Dr Tan Liok Ee
Bureau on Learning Difficulties
Penang Caring Society Complex
Rm. CO–3-GF, Jalan Utama
10 450 Pulau Pinang
Malaysia
Tel.: (604) 2278611
Email: boldplace@yahoo.com

Pn Sariah bt Amirin
The Kuala Lumpur Dyslexia Association
No. 6 Persiaran Kuantan
Off Jalan Kuantan
Titiwangsa, Setapak
53 200 Kuala Lumpur
Tel.: (603) 40255109

CHAPTER AUTHOR

Caroline Gomez
Jabatan Pendidikan
Fakulti Pengajian Pendidikan
Universiti Putra Malaysia
43 400 UPM Serdang
Selangor Darul Ehsan
Malaysia
Tel.: (603) 89468177
Email: cagomez@putra.upm.edu.my

DYSLEXIA IN MALTA

Christine Firman

INTRODUCTION

Malta is a small island which has two official languages: English and Maltese. The NMC (1999)[1] states that 'With regard to the official languages, all schools must adopt the policy of using two languages.' While most children seem to cope with the development of literacy skills in two languages, others, particularly dyslexics, are finding this extremely difficult. Unfortunately, opportunities for further education can be limited if a child fails to develop adequate competence. For example, at the age of 11+ most Maltese children sit a competitive examination in both English and Maltese. Failure in either of the two languages 'condemns' a child to a less academic secondary school. At secondary level, the equivalent of General Certificate of Secondary Education (GCSE) passes in Maltese and English are prerequisites for tertiary education and adequate employment. A dyslexic child is therefore obliged to study both languages since his or her horizons can otherwise be severely limited.

ATTITUDES TO DYSLEXIA

The attitude to dyslexia is now more positive. The Malta Dyslexia Association, established in 1985, has made many significant contributions. While until a few years ago it was considered to be a 'condition which existed overseas', today dyslexia is the concern of many Maltese professionals. Psychologists, speech therapists and social workers are aware of this problem and undergraduate teachers can attend a one-credit course on Specific Learning Difficulties (SpLD). Furthermore, practising teachers are given the opportunity of attending in-service training courses organized by the SpLD Service during the summer recess.

International Book of Dyslexia: A Guide to Practice and Resources. Edited by Ian Smythe, John Everatt and Robin Salter. ISBN 0-471-49646-4. © 2004 John Wiley & Sons, Ltd.

ASSESSMENT PROCEDURES

The bilingual situation can lead to a number of problems with assessments. To begin with, no standardized tests are available in Malta. English standardized measures are used both for intelligence quotient (IQ) testing and for investigating levels of literacy – attainment is discussed in terms of a British population though some allowances are made to cater for cultural differences. The situation with Maltese literacy is more problematic in that only one standardized reading test is available (Bartolo, 1988).[2] Having now worked in the field of dyslexia for a good number of years, it has been necessary to establish some more 'localized' criteria for the identification of dyslexia in Malta. It is more often than not a comparative investigation of the performance on such items as phonological awareness, single word reading, word spelling and non-word reading in the two languages which can give some reliable information about the nature of the problem the child is experiencing.

THE SPECIFIC LEARNING DIFFICULTIES SERVICE

In September 1997 the Specific Learning Difficulties Service was set up in the Education Division. This is a service which caters for all children in primary and secondary state, church and independent schools in Malta and Gozo. The service aims at developing awareness of the difficulties encountered by dyslexic individuals and offers consultation as to the management of the dyslexic child in class. The SpLD service now has a good amount of up-to-date teaching programmes and literacy resources which are not only appropriate for the dyslexic child but also for any child who might be experiencing literacy difficulties. Schools are starting to realize that the techniques advocated for the dyslexic child can benefit the whole school and for this reason staff administrators come to the Centre to investigate how they can improve literacy skills in the school situation. This, of course, is quite a recent and encouraging development – dyslexia is not looked upon as an isolated condition which no one wants to know about.

Apart from carrying out assessments and acting in a consultancy capacity with schools, the SpLD Service has also carried out some experimental reading courses to identify the most effective teaching techniques in our bilingual situation. The following is an overview of some of the most effective courses carried out by the SpLD Service.

REMEDIATION AND INTERVENTION

Some 36 children split into groups of 5 were included in the 6-week experimental reading course. They were 'ferried' into the SpLD Service in state-funded transport and received an hour and a half of intensive intervention twice a week.

Meeting other children who were experiencing the same kind of difficulties proved to be therapeutic. Children responded extremely well to multi-sensory teaching methods and much progress was noted. Their comments at the end of the course were somewhat unexpected – on being asked what they had learnt they said, 'New things like sounds and reading'. This is all the more surprising if one takes into consideration that the children had been exposed to teaching in two languages for at least four years and yet they had not developed the basic concepts of literacy.

Following the success of this first course a 12-week experimental course was held. This time a larger number of children was included hence the necessity to organize weekly courses over a longer period of time. Structured multi-sensory teaching was imparted to the different levels. While this second course was also effective and some good results were achieved, the increase in the number of weeks proved to be a negative factor. As time went by and the heat increased, the novelty of leaving schools and attending the Centre began to wane. It was generally felt that shorter but more intensive courses proved to be more effective.

The success of the first two courses led to even greater demands on the Education Department for more courses. A 'paired reading course' was organized. Assessments carried out by the SpLD Service were analysed and those who had gone beyond the initial stages of reading and were likely to benefit were invited to join. Parents attended a preliminary meeting. The nature of their commitment was stressed, they had to attend the Centre on a weekly basis to receive instruction on phonological awareness, spelling skills and paired reading techniques. Children were brought to the Centre on alternate weeks and in this way the SpLD staff, together with assistants, were able to ensure that the techniques were being implemented. At the end of the course, participants were re-tested and evaluation was carried out. Much progress was registered – children, parents and class teachers were amazed at what had been achieved as a result of structured multi-sensory teaching programmes.

CONCLUSION

While there is now more awareness of dyslexia in both state and private sectors, much work still has to be carried out with employers. As yet, adults still hesitate to discuss their learning problems, fearing that they might be misunderstood and their condition misinterpreted. It is hoped that in the next years the plight of the adult dyslexics will also improve.

NOTES

1 National Minimum Curriculum.
2 Maltese Word Reading Test, Test Construction Unit, Education Department, Malta.

REFERENCES

Bartolo, P.A. (1988) *Maltese Word Reading Test*. Malta: Test Construction Unit Education Dept.
Firman, C., Francica, C. and Grech, K. (2001) Paired reading and the dyslexic child – how effective? *Dyslexia Review*, 13 (1).

ORGANIZATIONS

The Dylexia Association
San Pawl Tat targa
Naxxar
NXR 06
Malta
Tel.: +356 41 33 05
Fax: +356 41 36 74

SpLD Service
The Mall
Floriana
Malta
Tel.: 0035621234965

CHAPTER AUTHOR

Christine Firman
SpLD Service
The Mall
Floriana
Malta
Email: christine.firman@gov.mt

DYSLEXIA IN NAMIBIA

Kazuvire Veii

INTRODUCTION

Through its mandate to provide education and training to all, including children with special needs, the Namibian Ministry of Basic Education has adopted a policy that guides it in its provision of services to children with special educational needs. Namibia's adopted policy is informed by the recent global educational reforms that have focused on education for all and inclusive education. Inclusive education has been premised on the understanding that all learners should be taken into account, embraced and considered as viable members of educational communities.

POLICY

The Ministry of Basic Education's policy on special education, and ultimately on learning disabilities including dyslexia, is executed by the Directorate of Special Education. Its objective is to provide assistance to impaired children or children with special needs as early as possible and to assist them to become fully integrated into society. The strategy is to achieve these objectives by integrating students with special needs into the regular educational programs (Mowes, 1997). As stated above, the policy on special education is supposed to inform the Ministry of Basic Education in its implementation of the special educational needs services. Unfortunately, despite the guiding policy, not much has been done to help children with special needs. First and foremost, unlike the UK and the USA, Namibia has neither an operational definition of nor diagnostic criteria for learning disabilities/difficulties, including dyslexia. In the absence of such a conceptualization, no proper or formal diagnosis of that disorder can be made. The lack of a formal diagnosis means that relevant, pertinent, and effective remedial services cannot be delivered to meet the needs of the individual child. Second, there is a severe shortage of psychologists in

International Book of Dyslexia: A Guide to Practice and Resources. Edited by Ian Smythe, John Everatt and Robin Salter. ISBN 0-471-49646-4. © 2004 John Wiley & Sons, Ltd.

Namibia, particularly educational/school psychologists. Therefore, there are no suitably qualified personnel to make formal diagnoses of learning disabilities (LD) among school-age children. As Mowes (1997) and Zimba (1999) report, over-burdened Namibian school teachers have very little or no specialized training in special education. As a result, they are not able to meet the needs of children with special educational needs in the classroom, let alone carry out a preliminary screening of possible LD.

PRACTICE

Although the Ministry of Basic Education has an obligation and a commitment to help children with special educational needs, it has a minimal number of institutions meant for such purposes. Children who have what seem to be genuine, conspicuous and obvious special educational needs are accommodated in these facilities. Children with learning difficulties also may be accommodated in these institutions. According to Mowes (1997), children are referred for special education if they have repeated the same grade twice or if a child has failed two grades consecutively. The reasons for such repeated failure are rarely considered. This being the case, the learning difficulties that lead to a child being sent to a special education facility are not operationally defined or informed by any theoretical perspective. Using such uninformed, unscientific criteria for referral and placement is an inadequate way of identifying children with LD. Children can potentially be misdiagnosed and wrongly categorized as being in need of special educational services (e.g., children who have missed large amounts of schooling). Additionally, a child who really does need such services may be placed in the wrong category of special needs. A child's poor academic performance may not necessarily be due to an LD. Other factors such as emotional problems, neglect, abuse, or a mere lack of motivation and interest may be the underlying factors contributing to a child's poor academic performance. Therefore, a referral for, or placement in, a special educational needs programme may not serve the purpose since the remedial services being provided may not be addressing and meeting the specific needs of those children who may be victims of misdiagnosis and misplacement.

Finally, physical facilities such as schools for special educational needs children are insufficient. Mowes (1997) reports, for example, that there are 21 schools for 375 children with LD in the Windhoek Central region and another five in the south region for 109 children. For the 375 LD children in the central region, there are 31 teachers, while the 109 children in the south are catered for by seven teachers. This gives us teacher–student ratios of between 1 : 12 and 1 : 16. Given the individual needs of such children, there is an obvious lack of facilities, as well as a lack of special education teachers. Additionally, the few available teachers are insufficiently trained to meet the needs of special students.

Hengari (1998) makes reference to learning problems being a challenge facing many Namibian teachers every day. He goes on to talk about various categories of students with learning problems including mental retardation, learning difficulties/disabilities, emotional, and behavioural disorders. Mowes (1997) makes a distinction between 'learning difficulties' and 'slight learning difficulties'. Neither Hengari nor Mowes inform the reader as to how these disorders are defined, what their diagnostic criteria are, who diagnoses them, and who decides on the right course of intervention. Given the fact that there are no suitably qualified personnel to carry out diagnoses and treatment, the validity of these categories and other psychological disorders that children are given may be questionable.

Although there is a lack of suitably qualified professionals to render the right type of services to the needy children of Namibia, there is the will to turn the situation around, at least on the part of the institutions of higher learning in Namibia. This is evident in the teacher training programmes at the University of Namibia and the teacher training colleges. These programmes include sensitizing the trainee teachers to children with special needs. To succeed, these programmes need the support, financial and otherwise, of the primary funding agent of education, namely, the Namibian government. The support of the student teachers in these training and educational programmes is also of great importance to ensure their success.

Inclusive education and teacher training programmes to educate the pre-service as well as in-service teachers have been put in place. This needs to be strengthened by developing a comprehensive, clear, and implementable policy on education of Namibian children with special needs because the current policy needs rethinking, revision, and enhancement (Zimba, 1999). While this is a good initiative which we all hope will gain momentum and eventually come to fruition, this is only part of the equation to solve the problem. In addition to policy formulation and teacher training, Namibia needs to embark upon a massive programme for training psychologists who will do their part in addressing the special educational needs of those affected children.

REFERENCES

Hengari, J.U. (1995) Reading difficulties expressed by Grade 1 learners in a primary school in Namibia: a contextual study. Unpublished MPhil thesis presented to the Institute of Education, University of Oslo.

Mowes, A. (1997) Policy and practices on the education of children with learning disabilities. Unpublished paper. Windhoek: Faculty of Education, University of Namibia.

Zimba, R.F. (1999) Inclusive education efforts at supporting the learning of Namibian students with special needs. In *Proceedings of the Workshop on Inclusive Education in Namibia: The Challenge for Teacher Education*, Rossing Foundation Center, Khomasdal, 24–26 March, 1999.

CHAPTER AUTHOR

Kazuvire Veii
Department of Psychology
University of Surrey
Guildford
GU2 7XH
United Kingdom
Email: k.veii@surrey.ac.uk

DYSLEXIA IN THE NETHERLANDS

Kees P. van den Bos

RESEARCH DEVELOPMENTS

As a continuation of Pieter Reitsma's excellent chapter on Dutch language, definition and dyslexia research developments (see Part I of this book), there is the following news. Since 1997 the Dutch National Science Foundation (NWO) has co-sponsored an ambitious dyslexia research programme 'Identifying the Core Features of Developmental Dyslexia: A Multidisciplinary Approach'. The programme is conducted by researchers from the Dutch universities of Amsterdam, Nijmegen, and Groningen. It addresses three themes. One theme is prospective longitudinal research. The neurocognitive development of a group of children at risk of familial dyslexia is followed from birth on and compared with a control group. These groups will be followed for ten years. The second theme is genetic research. Over 200 families with two or more dyslexic children will be studied. The third theme is early intervention and prevention. This theme is addressed by three related projects that are conducted from 2001 till 2004. Common to these three projects is the selection of 4-year-old children who are genetically at risk, i.e. they are from families in which at least one parent and one other close relative are dyslexic. Two-thirds of these at-risk children will participate in training experiments. The remaining one-third will comprise the no-training risk-control group. Furthermore, a control group of no-risk children will be added to the design. The children will be studied for four years. All three intervention projects will study the effects on later reading and spelling performance of a base programme that trains various aspects of phonological sensitivity and skill, and letter-sound learning. The projects differ in additional focus on: pre-reading learning and attention mechanisms (Project 1, Aryan van der Leij, University of Amsterdam), possible differential effects of natural speech versus synthetic speech conditions in the computerized phonology-intervention programme (Project 2, Ludo Verhoeven, University of Nijmegen), and possible differential effects of a rapid-naming training programme (involving alphanu-

International Book of Dyslexia: A Guide to Practice and Resources. Edited by Ian Smythe, John Everatt and Robin Salter. ISBN 0-471-49646-4. © 2004 John Wiley & Sons, Ltd.

meric and non-alphanumeric stimuli) compared to the phonological base programme (Project 3, Kees van den Bos, University of Groningen). Progress reports on these and other projects can be obtained from the Dutch National Science Foundation (NWO), which also issues the biannual *Dyslexia News Bulletin* and organizes lecture-and-information 'afternoons' at central places. The bulletin can be obtained from NWO-Onderzoeks-programma Dyslexie.

PROMOTING PUBLIC AWARENESS

Dyslexia is a regular theme in the Dutch media, including television (e.g., in 2001 there was a special programme *Nova*, presented by A. Van der Leij). Also see the NWO-efforts mentioned above. Other signs that the general public and students of education have a keen interest in dyslexia are the impressive sales figures of recent books on dyslexia, such as those by A. van der Leij (1998), J. Sas and C. Wieringa (1998), J.H. Loonstra and F. Schalkwijk (1999) and Tom Braams (2002).

THE PARENT ASSOCIATION

The National Parent Association for Developmental, Behavioural, and Learning Problems, with almost 20,000 members is called Balans. Balans frequently organizes national and regional conferences, meetings and workshops. They issue a highly informative bimonthly journal (*Balans Belang*; chief editor Arga Paternotte) and brochures and books.

THE NETHERLANDS DYSLEXIA ASSOCIATION

The Stichting Dyslexie Nederland (SDN) (Netherlands Dyslexia Association, NDA) was founded in 1983 by the late Professor Joep J. Dumont of the University of Nijmegen. The association is formed of representatives of the scientific community and practitioners in the field of special education. The association's objective is to enhance the scientific quality of diagnosis and treatment of dyslexia as practised in the Netherlands. This is done through publication of proposals of protocols pertaining to the issue of management of dyslexia and by disseminating scientific knowledge through national conferences and experts meetings.

ENHANCEMENT OF PROFESSIONAL SKILLS: SCREENING, DIAGNOSIS, AND TREATMENT PROTOCOLS

The NDA recently issued the booklet *Dyslexia: Classification, Diagnosis, and Dyslexia Declaration* (Van der Leij *et al.*, 2000). The declaration is a document, to be issued by a certified psychologist after psychological assessment following the association's protocol, declaring a person to be dyslexic. The NDA defines dyslexia as 'a disorder characterized by enduring problems in the automatization of word identification (reading) and/or spelling'. A dyslexia declaration is based on three complementary types of diagnoses. In accordance with the DSM-IV approach, the first type is classificatory with a set of norm and impairment-referenced criteria to be met. Next, hypotheses must be formulated, stating possible cognitive and biological cause(s). Finally, guidelines must be given for treatment. This part focuses on the 'broader picture' of the person with dyslexia. That is, the person's educational context, learning perspectives (home and school) and psycho-social functioning are described. Furthermore, implications of possible co-morbidity of other disorders, such as AD(H)D, and impairment of other areas of learning, such as language and communication, mathematics, etc., are indicated. Finally, a treatment plan, including the necessary facilities at school or work, is part of the dyslexia declaration. In the past two years, a considerably expanded version of the 2000 booklet containing elaborations on theory, operationalization, and educational planning has been prepared by the NDA's board members and invited specialists, and this version (under the title *Handleiding Diagnose Dyslexie* [Manual of Diagnosis of Dyslexia] by A. van der Leij *et al.*) will be published soon. A few months after the NDA-issued booklet, another important dyslexia protocol was distributed to thousands of schools in the Netherlands, entitled *Protocol leesproblemen en dyslexie* [Protocol reading problems and dyslexia] and written by H. Wentink and L. Verhoeven (2000). It is focused on early elementary grades, and provides detailed information on screening and treatment steps to be taken by teachers and remedial specialists. A protocol for higher elementary grades is in preparation. Similarly, the booklet *Dyslexie, een praktische gids voor scholen voor voortgezet onderwijs* [Dyslexia: A practical guide for secondary schools] authored by Heleen Schoots and the national Catholic Educational Center (KPC) was published in 2002 by the Dutch Ministry of Education, Culture, and Sciences. Also this booklet will be followed by a more detailed protocol.

LEGISLATION, POLICIES AND RESPONSIBILITY

Currently, there are only two law-enforced provisions that can be 'claimed' by dyslexic persons at various stages of secondary education. Based on Article 85a, second section, of the Law on Secondary Education, a school can ask the central government for extra financial support in order to let the dyslexic person participate in a remedially oriented programme. Second, the statutory order on final examinations allows the dyslexic pupil to spend an extra 30 minutes to complete a particular test. From a recent article in the journal *Balans Belang* (no. 59, 1999), it is clear that schools differ widely with regard to their understanding and management of dyslexia. It is strongly recommended that all schools make their dyslexia policy explicit. All teachers in a school and the dyslexic students and their parents should be able to refer to a clear and concrete dyslexia policy which would describe formal and informal treatment procedures, facilities, rights and duties of all parties involved.

PLATFORM DYSLEXIE NEDERLAND (PLATFORM DYSLEXIA IN THE NETHERLANDS]

An exciting new development seems to be the recent establishment of an 'overarching' association, namely, the Platform Dyslexie Nederland. The PDN's central aim is to promote as integrated and broadly supported policy with regard to the many aspects of dyslexia in a life-span perspective. There is some overlap with the goals of the NDA, but in its presentation the PDN operates differently by promoting 'business plans' and working groups for each of the sectors: lobby or pressure groups, universities and teacher colleges (e.g., Hogeschool Windesheim at Zwolle, Fontys Hogescholen at Tilburg, and Seminarium voor Orthopedagogiek at Utrecht), and school support organizations, and provides financing of help (including advice to health insurance companies), etc. Finally, the PDN listens very carefully to dyslexic persons themselves. For example, a key person in the PDN is Balt van Raamsdonk, severely dyslexic himself, and since he retired from business, fully devoted to bringing the topic of dyslexia back to where it belongs in the first place: the school!

WHERE TO GO FOR HELP?

A very informative site is http://www.dyslexie.nl. This site also has a link with adult-support organizations, such as Woortblind (www.woortblind.myweb.nl).

All Dutch schools for primary education are supported by Regional Institutions for Educational Services. Several institutions have opened dyslexia offices, some with sites on the Internet, e.g. www.dyslexiecentrumpravoo.nl.

The parent association Balans has a help desk that can be contacted on Monday, Tuesday, Wednesday, or Thursday mornings at tel. +31 900 202 0065.

There are also numerous private institutes, many of which are known by the NDA members and Balans. NDA members can be contacted through Balans.

REFERENCES

Braams, T. (2002) *Dyslexie: een complex taalproblem.* [Dyslexia: A complex language problem.] Amsterdam: Boom.

Loonstra, J.H. and Schalkwijk, F. (eds) (1999) *Omgaan met dyslexie: Sociale en emotionele aspecten.* [Handling dyslexia: Socio-emotional aspects.] Leuven/Apeldoorn: Garant.

Sas, J. and Wieringa, C. (1998) *Leesmoeilijkheden.* [Reading difficulties.] Groningen: Wolters-Noordhoff.

Van der Leij, A. (1998) *Leesproblemen.* [Reading problems.] Rotterdam: Lemniscaat.

Van der Leij, A., Struiksma, A.J.C. and Ruijssenaars, A.J.J.M. (2000) *Dyslexia: Classification, Diagnosis and Dyslexia Definition.* Bilthoven: Stichting Dyslexie Nederland (NDA, Balans).

Wentink, H. and Verhoeven, L. (2000) *Protocol Leesproblemen en dyslexie.* [Protocol reading problems and dyslexia.] Nijmegen: Expertisecentrum Nederlands.

ORGANIZATIONS

Balans
De Kwinkelier 39
3722 AR Bilthoven
or Postbus 93
3720 AB Bilthoven
Tel.: +31 30 225 5050
Fax: +31 30 225 2440
Email: Arga.Paternotte@balansdigitaal.nl

NWO-Onderzoeksprogramma Dyslexie
Postbus 93138
The Hague
Tel.: +31 70 3440757
Email: dyslexie@nwo.nl

CHAPTER AUTHOR

Kees P. van den Bos
Special Education Section
University of Groningen
Grote Rozenstraat 38
9712 TJ Groningen
The Netherlands
Tel.: +31 50 363 65 89
Fax: 31 50 363 65 64
Email: K.P.van.den.Bos@ppsw.rug.nl

DYSLEXIA IN NEW ZEALAND

James Hawkins

INTRODUCTION

In New Zealand there continues to be only a limited awareness of dyslexia as a specific and significant difficulty. The Ministry of Education does not officially recognize dyslexia, the Reading Recovery programme does not recognize it, and nor do the Specialist Education Service Psychologists. Most schools and teachers do not think of dyslexia as a real entity. This is not surprising because the Colleges of Education, which train teachers, do not provide any training about dyslexia. In the last two years new positions in the schooling system have been created for teachers with responsibility for children with 'moderate learning and behavioural needs'. A small number of these teachers are attached to a cluster of several schools, under the control of the school principals. These teachers are called 'resource teachers of learning and behaviour'. Although dyslexia is not officially included in their job description, it is very likely that children with dyslexia will be referred to these teachers because of the learning difficulties that they will show.

LEGISLATION AND POLICY

There is no legislation or government policy that specifically names or addresses dyslexia. However, there is a provision under the New Zealand Qualifications Authority (which controls and monitors qualifications and examinations) for the use of a 'reader-writer' for students with an established learning disability. Dyslexia, if diagnosed by a professional such as an educational psychologist, qualifies a student for a reader-writer.

INDEPENDENT SUPPORT

In New Zealand the major area of support for those with dyslexia is non-governmental community groups. They do not receive funding from the government and have to raise

International Book of Dyslexia: A Guide to Practice and Resources. Edited by Ian Smythe, John Everatt and Robin Salter. ISBN 0-471-49646-4. © 2004 John Wiley & Sons, Ltd.

funds through applications to groups that support charitable organizations, and through basic fund-raising by the members of their organization. These groups provide assessments and access to private, part-time tutoring which is usually outside school hours. Sometimes the private tutoring occurs at school, during school hours but this is at the discretion of the school, and is the exception rather than the rule. Most of these groups offer some kind of course for teachers, as teachers do not get any training about dyslexia as pre-service training, or in-service training.

At the tertiary level of education (university and polytechnics), there is some recognition of dyslexia. Most of these have 'Learning Centres' which provide help for tertiary students with learning difficulties, and some of them recognize dyslexia.

PROFESSIONAL AWARENESS

Professional awareness of dyslexia is also at a low level in New Zealand, because it is not officially part of the policy of the government in relation to special needs in schools. There is no strong culture of acceptance of dyslexia. Dyslexia is a term used in the public domain, and is recognized by the public as a condition, but there is limited understanding and knowledge of exactly what dyslexia is. There is no legislation or official provision for adults with dyslexia.

In the past three to five years there have been seminars, conferences, and publicity about dyslexia which have raised public awareness about dyslexia. Courses for teachers and teacher aides have been run by community groups which include dyslexia. In general, there is now a much better awareness of dyslexia, but there is still no official recognition, or provision in the schooling system. There is still a long way to go, but progress is taking place.

ORGANIZATIONS

Learning Difficulties Coalition of New Zealand
PO Box 6748
Wellington
New Zealand
Tel.: (04) 3828944
Email: ldc@paradise.net.nz
Website: www.ldc.co.nz

Learning Difficulties Coalition of Auckland Charitable Trust
PO Box 503
Warkworth
Auckland
New Zealand
Tel.: 080064 5322

Dyslexia Association of Wellington
Box 11953
Wellington
New Zealand
Tel.: 035226 5747

Seabrook McKenzie Centre
68 London Street
Christchurch
New Zealand
Tel.: (03) 381 5383

SPELD NZ
Head Office
c/o Secretary
PO Box 25
Dargaville
Tel.: 09-439-5955
Email: faj@xtra.co.nz
Website: www.speld.org.nz/contact.html

CHAPTER AUTHOR

James Hawkins
SPELD New Zealand Inc
PO Box 27
122 Wellington
New Zealand

Dyslexia in North Cyprus

Ersin Öztoycan and Catherine Martin

INTRODUCTION

It was necessity that led to the creation of the North Cyprus Dyslexia Association (NCDA). Personal experience showed there was little understanding of dyslexia and even worse promotion on the island of those who have specific learning difficulties. Faced with the practical realities of the situation and motivated by the European Dyslexia Association and the Scottish Dyslexia Association, the NCDA was established in 2001 to work towards raising awareness and understanding of dyslexia among the general public.

AWARENESS RAISING

To this end, and in conjunction with a local education authority, the NCDA organized a number of seminars throughout the island targeting 'in service' training of primary school teachers with regard to the signs and symptoms of dyslexia.

Interest was extremely encouraging, which prompted the organization of an awareness raising conference in October 2002, at which guest speakers Dr Ürman Korkmazlar of Istanbul medical faculty and Dr Gavin Reid of Edinburgh University shared their expertise in the field with an enthusiastic and interested audience, some of whom were able to avail themselves of the follow-up workshops given by the visiting academics. These workshops concentrated on the practicability and importance of recognizing personality traits and learning styles when devising remedial learning programmes for students with specific learning difficulties. Feedback from the conference and workshops was positive: our initial aim of raising awareness and highlighting dyslexia had been achieved.

Clearly it was now a case of 'What next?' A number of strategies and initiatives are already in place, due in the main to the funding provided through the United Nations Office of Project Services (UNOPS) for a project called 'Assistance for those affected by

International Book of Dyslexia: A Guide to Practice and Resources. Edited by Ian Smythe, John Everatt and Robin Salter. ISBN 0-471-49646-4. © 2004 John Wiley & Sons, Ltd.

dyslexia'. Furthermore, under the auspices of the Ministry of Education, early November 2002 saw the opening of the North Cyprus Dyslexia Centre.

The centre will provide professional help, accurate information and advisory services for parents, students, teachers and other professionals. This service will be given in a confidential manner by a small professional screening and remedial support team for students. These are early days and so far the indications are very favourable. Interest in and awareness of dyslexia have been raised. Returned questionnaires after the conference and workshops overwhelmingly requested back-up visits to schools, more information and a very genuine desire to move forward.

THE WAY AHEAD

What is undoubtedly needed now and indeed is essential for progress is the instigation of a research programme that will examine the problems specific to our first language and bilingual community. To our knowledge, there is little or no research to draw upon which deals with the learning and teaching of Turkish to those affected by dyslexia. The fact that there is little research known to us presents a number of problems. Essentially we have no unmodified assessment battery with which we can assess students. All existing materials are flawed in that there can be no meaningful direct translation because of the structure of the Turkish language, i.e. phonetic and suffix. We feel that such research would be of immense value, not only to our specific needs, but also to the wider 'dyslexia' community.

From our initial findings we are certain that this area of research would be a major step forward, for although we are managing adequately with the materials available, it does lead one to question if assessment could be more accurate using materials which had been developed with our specific language needs in mind. Although there has been increased interest in this area of research, as yet we do not have a universally acceptable useful multi-language battery of assessment materials at our disposal.

Interest in our initial campaign has been overwhelming, and we approach our next steps with a mixture of emotions. First, we remain incredibly enthusiastic; second, in truth, a little overwhelmed by the task ahead. However, where there's a will, there's a way! The North Cyprus Dyslexia Association will find a way forward to assist the children and adults, parents, teachers and community to understand and positively accommodate dyslexia. We look forward to the time when dyslexia in North Cyprus will not be considered a learning difficulty but rather just another learning difference.

ORGANIZATION

Kuzey Kilris Disleksi Dernegi (North Cyprus Dyslexia Association)
Yeni Organize Sanay
Bolgesi
Leifkosa
Mersin 10
Turkey
Tel: +90 392 234 6870
Email: dyslexia_ncda@hotmail.com

CHAPTER AUTHORS

Ersin Öztoycan
Chairperson, NCDA

Catherine Martin
Educational communications coordinator, NCDA
Yeni Organize Sanay
Bolgesi
Leifkosa
Mersin 10
Turkey

DYSLEXIA IN NORWAY

Berit Bogetvedt

PUBLIC AWARENESS

In general, the Norwegian people are quite familiar with the term 'dyslexia' and what it means. Dyslexia has gradually become a well-known word through the media and information at school and elsewhere. Although most people do not know the exact reasons why the handicap arises, or the biological facts of dyslexia, they tend to be acquainted with the phenomenon and what problems it causes for those affected by it.

PROFESSIONAL AWARENESS

Teachers are expected to know about dyslexia and to recognize the signs of dyslexia in the pupils. Especially at elementary school level, this is considered important. What happens in practice, however, can be quite a different story. The Norwegian Dyslexia Association is often told about teachers who have practically no knowledge of the topic, and they are thus unable to recognize the signs of dyslexia when these are seen in class. This is a problem and the Association is very busy sending information material to elementary and secondary schools around the country in order to prevent this.

ASSESSMENT METHODS

Psychologists/pedagogues in the Pedagogical Psychological Service are responsible for assessing both children and adults. Giving children priority, they use mostly standardized tests. In cases where the child has been diagnosed as dyslexic, the psychologist/pedagogue recommends special education and individual education plans for the child, which the school ought to follow.

International Book of Dyslexia: A Guide to Practice and Resources. Edited by Ian Smythe, John Everatt and Robin Salter. ISBN 0-471-49646-4. © 2004 John Wiley & Sons, Ltd.

LEGISLATION, POLICIES AND RESPONSIBILITY

All schoolchildren with a dyslexia diagnosis are entitled by law to be taught in accordance with their special, individual needs. A separate educational plan is to be worked out by professionals in co-operation with the parents, as soon as the diagnosis has been confirmed. The special teaching is guaranteed by law until the pupil has finished upper secondary school, normally at the age of 18 years.

Dyslexic pupils can apply to a special office in their region to borrow a computer, which they can use at home and/or at school. Many children now use computers and find it most useful in their learning process. The school is in charge of buying the right computer programs. The computer may also be used in the various examinations. Other means of help are audio books and tape recorders. These are used when found appropriate for the pupil's needs and are also subject to the school's acceptance.

At university level, dyslexics have far less guaranteed rights than at school. They are considered adults and thus other rules apply. Universities and colleges are not obliged by law to consider the needs of dyslexic students. However, most of them take these problems seriously and have worked out individual guidelines to make it easier for dyslexics to study. Examples of these internal rules are extended time at examinations, permission to use computers in examinations, and dyslexics can also often attach an anonymous confirmation of their handicap to their essay in order to inform their examiner about their spelling problems.

ADULT PROVISION

This year the authorities responsible for the labour market plan to give special focus to, among others, adult dyslexics. Whether this will actually be of any help for job-seeking dyslexics remains to seen.

BILINGUALISM

Today there is a growing awareness of the problem of dyslexia for bilingual children. Tests and training programmes are being developed, but the work of implementing these has just started.

ORGANIZATION

Dysleksiforbundet i Norge
Box 8731 Youngstorget
0028 Oslo
Norway
Tel.: +47 22 47 4450
Email: post@dysleksiforbundet.no

CHAPTER AUTHOR

Berit Bogetvedt
Sknarpsnogata
3530 Royse
Norway

DYSLEXIA IN THE PHILIPPINES

Dina Ocampo

INTRODUCTION

The Philippines, which has an estimated population of 72 million, is a multilingual country that has around 75 major languages and over 500 dialects (Rubrico, 1997). The majority of these dialects have evolved from a dominant language with greater regional influence such as Cebuano, Bicol, Hiligaynon, Pangasinan, Pampango, Waray-Samarnon, Tagalog, and Ilocano. Filipino children learn one of these languages/dialects first because it is spoken within the geographic area in which they live. As they grow up, they learn other languages or dialects that are similar to the one they already speak. Thus, it is highly unlikely to find a Filipino who speaks only one language. Most Filipinos speak more than three languages including their mother tongue. Among these will be Filipino, and English.

NATIONAL LANGUAGE

Filipino (formerly Pilipino) evolved from Tagalog, which in 1935 was legislated as the national language. Tagalog is a member of the Malayan (or Western) branch of the Malayo-Polynesian linguistic family. Due to trade and colonization, numerous other languages have influenced Tagalog. Four decades later in 1973, Pilipino replaced Tagalog, which was perceived as a regional language that not all Filipino people could understand and learn. Filipino is now the national language that has developed on the basis of existing Philippine and other languages (Constitution of the Republic of the Philippines, 1987). Therefore, Filipino, as it is used now, can best be described as an amalgamation of Tagalog, English, Spanish, Sanskrit, Arabic, Chinese and the other widely spoken Philippines languages. It is the first language of about 55 per cent of Filipinos. Since it is one of the languages of instruction and of popular media (i.e. films, and television) most people eventually learn it.

International Book of Dyslexia: A Guide to Practice and Resources. Edited by Ian Smythe, John Everatt and Robin Salter. ISBN 0-471-49646-4. © 2004 John Wiley & Sons, Ltd.

THE FILIPINO ALPHABET

In its present form, Filipino is composed of 28 letters, which have the same names as the English alphabet. It is a transparent orthography that shares all 26 letters of the English alphabet plus an additional two letters (ñ and ng). Originally it had 20 letters (a, b, k, d, e, g, h, i, l, m, n, ng, o, p, r, s, t, u, w, y). It incorporates one letter from Spanish (ñ) and seven letters from the English alphabet (c, f, j, q, v, x, z) because numerous words in Filipino are words adapted from these two languages. Roman letters which the Spaniards introduced during the colonization period replaced the original orthography called the Baybayin (or Alibata). The orthography is nearly completely transparent.

The present phonology of Filipino has five vowel sounds and 23 consonants, all of which are found in or similar to the phonology of English. Filipino vowels and consonants are articulated distinctly so that when speaking, all the letters in a word can be heard. For example, in the Filipino word *tao* ('person') the two vowels are pronounced separately as ta-o where the letter 'a' sounds like the 'a' in *apple* and the letter 'o' sounds like the 'o' in *toe*. The vowels are also more akin to the short vowel sounds in English. For example, the Filipino word *anak* ('child') is spoken as [ä-näk] using approximately the same vowel sound that is used in the English word 'apple'.

The Philippines has one of the largest groups of English-speaking people in the world. English is an official language used widely in government, the popular media, law, commercial contexts and in education where it is used as a medium of instruction. Like most bilingual peoples, Filipinos code-switch extensively. 'Taglish' is frequently used in oral discourse. Words and phrases from English and Filipino are interspersed in sentences, especially in informal situations.

THE EDUCATIONAL CONTEXT

Mandated in the constitution of the Philippines is compulsory and free basic education. Public or free education is provided by the government, which is duty-bound to provide all children with access to schools or to instruction. Most Filipino children attend the public school system that offers ten years of schooling composed of six grades in elementary school and four years in secondary school. Private or fee-paying schools usually add two levels (kindergarten/preparatory and seventh grade) in the elementary school ladder, providing a total of 12 years of basic education. The Department of Education sets the minimum learning competencies that schools must ensure children attain and supervises both public and private schools. However, this government agency does not impose specific methods of instruction nor prescribe materials to be used in schools.

BILINGUAL EDUCATION

A feature of the Philippine educational system is its bilingual education policy. This aims for all students in Philippine schools to achieve competence in both Filipino and English through the teaching of both languages and their use as media of instruction at all levels. Therefore, children are taught to read and write in Filipino and English at the same time when they enter the formal school system in Grade I. In many regions of the Philippines, especially those near urban centres, children will have been immersed in the bilingual context from a very early age.

However, there are also many areas in the country that remain geographically isolated and do not have ease of access to the media. There are also areas where the dialect is based on another dominant language quite different from Tagalog. The children in these places would have little experience of either Filipino or English. In such contexts, the policy recommends that the child's first language be used as the initial language of literacy and to use it to bridge understanding of Filipino and English.

The bilingual education policy is implemented by teaching specific subjects in the curriculum in a specific language. Filipino is used to teach Filipino literature and language, social studies/social sciences, music, arts, physical education, home economics, practical arts and character education. English is used to teach science, mathematics, technology and English literature and language subjects.

SPECIAL NEEDS LEGISLATION

The Philippines has no specific legislation on dyslexia. It has broader laws that set the framework which guide the formulation of national strategies and programmes. The two most relevant laws that pertain to disability are the Child and Youth Welfare Code of 1974 and the Magna Carta for Disabled Persons (1992).

The law with the broader scope is the Child and Youth Welfare Code (Presidential Decree No. 603, 1974) which states that: 'every child has the right to an education commensurate with his abilities and to the development of his skills for the improvement of his capacity for service for himself and to his fellowmen'.

Public and private schools are encouraged to organize special classes for disabled children who come under the following categories: mentally retarded, physically handicapped, emotionally disturbed and children with severe mental illness. Unfortunately, there is no direct reference to children with dyslexia and other learning difficulties in the policies that have been formulated.

More recently, the Magna Carta for Disabled Persons (1992) has presented a slightly broader view of disabled persons. The special needs named in the Child and Youth Welfare Code were revised to include the phrase 'other types of exceptional children'. Furthermore, this new law requires the government to ensure that quality special education is available and that it is unlawful for any learning institution to deny a disabled person admission to any course it offers by reason of handicap or disability.

The change in terminology in the two laws shows that there has been a change in the understanding of special needs and disabilities. The definitions are broader, thus allowing for the inclusion of different learning needs and the development of new, more specialized educational provisions.

EDUCATIONAL AND FAMILY SUPPORT FOR CHILDREN WITH DYSLEXIA

Although there is a lack of legislation and explicit government support for children with dyslexia, there are non-governmental organizations whose mission is to push for the identification, teaching and inclusion of children and persons with dyslexia. In the past 15 years, an increasing number of parents and teachers have become concerned about children who demonstrate difficulties in learning to read and spell. More often than not, they try to find solutions to help children learn better. Most of the time, the teaching and training initiatives come from the Wordlab School and the Philippine Dyslexia Foundation (PDF). An affiliate of the International Dyslexia Association, the PDF is composed of parents, and teachers and aims to generate awareness and knowledge about dyslexia; to support families with dyslexic children; and to collaborate with government so that dyslexia may be recognized as a special need across the educational system (Ocampo, 1997).

IDENTIFICATION AND ASSESSMENT

Psychologists and developmental paediatricians assess children for dyslexia using the traditional intelligence tests. Most of these assessments use the discrepancy criteria between intelligence quotient (IQ) and achievement in distinguishing dyslexia from other learning issues.

Reading specialists assess children for reading difficulty using reading tests in English, diagnostic teaching and dyslexia screening tests. Assessment in Filipino is rarely done since standardized tests in Filipino are not available (Paterno and Ocampo-Cristobal, 1993).

Access to assessment is not always easy. Parents of children who cannot afford to bear the costs of assessment are unlikely to prioritize the assessment over the needs of the rest of the family. There are some foundations and institutions that significantly reduce the cost of assessment services for families in financial difficulties by offering subsidized fees as well or by enlisting the help of student interns in psychology, school counselling or education to conduct some aspects of the assessment process.

TEACHING

Children with dyslexia who are in regular education are basically supported by their parents. In most cases, the children receive individual teaching support from reading specialists which the families pay for privately.

Another alternative for the dyslexic child is the Wordlab School, the only school in the Philippines for children with dyslexia. Its curriculum is based on the view that dyslexia is a condition that results in a different way of learning which causes difficulty in learning to read, spell and write. The Wordlab School aims to provide quality elementary education for children with dyslexia. The school has adapted the Orton-Gillingham and Slingerland methods and developed a multi-sensory method of teaching literacy in Filipino and English. The curriculum has a very challenging content and is enriched by the direct instruction of study strategies and organizational skills. The teachers are subject area specialists who address each content area as though it were a reading lesson to encourage the application of literacy abilities in the different areas of learning.

In the past five years, children have moved on from the Wordlab School and back into mainstream education. More private schools in the country have been accepting and including children with dyslexia in regular classes. Some schools are starting to develop teaching support programmes for the children (Ocampo, 1995). Though this is a great improvement from the situation 15 years ago, most if not all of these children are in private education.

THE WAY AHEAD

Different pathways must be taken to achieve a widespread educational atmosphere that is friendly to and supportive of children with dyslexia in the Philippines. Among the more direct routes to this goal are a focus on teacher education, and collaborative work with education agencies in and outside of government.

Allocating state resources for research and programme development within the public school system is also of prime importance. This will create access to teaching support for more children who otherwise will remain unidentified and on the verge of failure in school. Conducting basic research on the incidence of dyslexia and other literacy-based difficulties which Filipino children experience is one concrete measure that must be urgently undertaken. A clearer understanding of the way dyslexia manifests among children who are bilingual or multilingual will provide a basis for the development of intervention programmes and assessment tools. Such research should also feed into the pre-service teacher education curricula so that future generations of teachers will be better equipped with knowledge and strategies to help children who experience literacy difficulties.

Wider-reaching awareness campaigns geared towards parents, professionals who work with children (i.e. medical doctors, speech therapists, psychologists, teachers) and policy-makers will likewise create greater access to support for more children, their families and schools. Finally, efforts to provide support for adults with dyslexia must be initiated. Higher education institutions should articulate systems by which persons with dyslexia can succeed in tertiary or continuing education.

REFERENCES

Almario, Virgilio S. (1997) 'Mulang Tagalog hanggang Filipino.' *Daluyan*. VIII (1–2). Quezon City: Sentro ng Wikang Pilipino, University of the Philippines System.

The Constitution of the Republic of the Philippines, 1987.

Ocampo, D. (1995) Individualized reading instruction for children with LD: the Wordlab Experience. *RAP Journal*, Silver Jubilee issue, 62–68.

Ocampo, D. (1997) Dyslexia in the Philippines. In R. Salter and I. Smythe (eds), *The International Book of Dyslexia*. London: World Dyslexia Network Foundation.

Paterno, M.E. and Ocampo-Cristobal, D. (1993) *Now What Do I Do? A Guide for Parents with Special Children*. Manila: Cacho Publishing House.

P.D. 603 (1974) Child and Youth Welfare Code, amended 1981, Republic of the Philippines.

Republic Act 7277 (1992) Magna Carta for Disabled Persons, Republic of the Philippines.

Rubrico, J.G.U. (1997) An annotated bibliography of works and studies on the history, structure, and lexicon of the cebuano language: 1610 to 1996. Unpublished thesis, University of the Philippines, Diliman, Quezon City.

ORGANIZATION

Wordlab School
28 7th Street
New Manila
Quezon City
Metro Manila
Phone: +632 7243871
Email: phil_dyslexia_foundation@hotmail.com

CHAPTER AUTHOR

Dina Ocampo
Reading Education Area
College of Education
University of the Philippines
1101 Diliman
Quezon City
The Philippines
Email: d.ocampo@up.edu.ph

DYSLEXIA IN POLAND

Marta Bogdanowicz

INTRODUCTION

Our concept of specific difficulties in reading and writing (developmental dyslexia) is based upon several general theories. These include Luria's (1976) theory of the functional organization of higher mental functions, Konorski's theory of integrative activity of the brain (1969), Tomaszewski's theory of action (1963) and Spionek's theory of psychomotor developmental deficits (1965). In accordance with these ideas, it has been accepted that reading and writing are highly structured psychological functions. They have a systematic structure and dynamic character (changeable in the process of learning). These complex functions are realized by the integrated activities of several brain areas. Their disturbances are usually defined as 'developmental dyslexia'. In the international classifications of diseases ICD-10 and DSM-IV, they are referred to as 'reading disturbances' and 'specific reading disturbances'. They are accompanied by the difficulties in learning how to write, in spite of normal intelligence, lack of sensory disturbances and normal environmental conditions – proper care of family and school.

Developmental dyslexia is treated in Poland as a syndrome consisting of three kinds of disturbances: specific reading difficulties (dyslexia), difficulties in spelling (dysorthography) and handwriting (dysgraphy). These are the result of disturbances in phonological and visual processing in time and space, which is observed as a narrow range of disturbances of psychomotor development of some cognitive functions (i.e. visual, auditory perception and memory, phonological skills and awareness), motor functions and their integration (perceptive-motor integration) (Bogdanowicz, 1987, 1997; Krasowicz-Kupis, 1997, 1999). These terms were based on the definitions accepted by the World Neurologists Conference in Boston in 1968 and the International Dyslexia Association in 1994.

International Book of Dyslexia: A Guide to Practice and Resources. Edited by Ian Smythe, John Everatt and Robin Salter. ISBN 0-471-49646-4. © 2004 John Wiley & Sons, Ltd.

HISTORY OF KNOWLEDGE OF DYSLEXIA IN POLAND

In Poland 'legastenia' has been known since after the First World War, when the first publications on this subject appeared by Sterling (1924–25), Bychowski (1934–35), Uzdańska
(1937) and Baley (1938). But it was Drath's (1959) article 'Dyslexia' which popularized
the new terminology. At that time she led multi-disciplinary work on therapeutic help for
dyslexic children with the staff of the Mental Hygiene and Psychiatry Institute of the Polish
Science Academy. In the University of Warsaw Spionek's work was of major significance,
as she adapted and popularized in Poland the basic set of diagnostic methods developed
in France. In 1965 the first monograph dealing with the psychomotor development of children and their difficulties in reading and writing was published in our country. This, as
well as the later monographs, summed up the investigations of Spionek (1965, 1973) and
her team. This in turn led to the development of different forms of treatment of dyslexic
children.

An educational therapeutic system of working with dyslexic children was created in the
form of correction-compensation exercises. It was developed from original techniques for
children with difficulties in learning designed by Magnuska in 1948. In 1959 Zakrzewska
and Markiewicz introduced a programme of 'double track rehabilitation' of dyslexic children consisting of two components: (1) psychomotor rehabilitation involving exercises in
visual, auditory perception and motor skills; and (2) psycho-education rehabilitation comprising various methods of improving reading and writing skills. In the 1960s the team at
the Outpatient Clinic for Neurotic Children in Gdansk (Bogdanowicz et al., 1969) started
to do research and therapeutic work in this field. Bogdanowicz popularized terms: 'developmental dyslexia' as a name for the syndrome of specific reading and writing difficulties; dyslexia, which includes 'dyslexia', 'dysorthography', and 'dysgraphy' (1969, 1983);
'children at risk of dyslexia' (1993); and 'perceptive-motor integration'(1987). She developed some methods of diagnosis and therapy e.g. the Good Start Method modelled on the
French Le Bon Départ method (Bogdanowicz 1986, 1987). In the 1970s therapeutic groups
were organized in most primary schools for work with dyslexic children after classes. The
first handbook for remedial teaching was published in Poland in 1976 by Zakrzewska.
Since then other guides for remedial teaching have been published. In 1994 the first guide
for parents and teachers was published by Bogdanowicz (On Dyslexia – Questions and
Answers to Parents and Teachers, modelled on the late Marion Welchman's booklet) and
is particularly popular. Since 1984 she and her team at the University of Gdansk have
organized 18 all-Polish conferences on difficulties in language, reading and writing in
which groups of foreign scientists and practitioners have taken part. In 1990 the Polish
Dyslexia Association was founded by Bogdanowicz and played an important role in developing the awareness of these problems in Polish society. Up until then the awareness of
dyslexia was still the domain of professionals working in psychological-education clinics
for children and adolescents, and some school teachers.

AWARENESS OF DYSLEXIA IN POLAND

In 1996 a survey was conducted to mark the 100th anniversary of research on dyslexia
and the 5th anniversary of the Polish Dyslexia Association (PDA). Its results indicated
that the term 'dyslexia' is presently quite well known in Poland (87 per cent of the 514

tested persons were familiar with it, 75 per cent believed they could define it).[1] Even though the word 'dyslexia' was familiar, knowledge was limited. The awareness of dyslexia was confined mainly to psychologists, educators and speech therapists employed in the clinics. The next best informed group was parents of dyslexic pupils, who were better informed than teachers. Different groups of teachers showed the same low level of understanding of the problems of dyslexia. Teachers of foreign languages had a very poor level of knowledge. The lowest level of awareness was shown by paediatricians and medical students (Bogdanowicz, 1997). This lack of knowledge is due to lack of appropriate teaching at the universities. Medical students who are preparing to be 'family doctors' in the future have no opportunity to learn anything about this matter during their six years of studies. Therefore the psychologists tend to educate themselves after graduating from the university. For over 30 years teachers have had the opportunity to be trained on special courses on remedial teaching organized by Teacher Training Centres, following which they can obtain a diploma and the title 'teacher therapist'. The need for the good preparation of professionals is evidenced by the high percentage of dyslexic children. Since 1994 the PDA has provided courses for teachers, other professionals and parents on how to help the dyslexic child at home.

The campaigns by the PDA have improved the awareness of dyslexia in our society. In 1993, 2001 and 2002 the PDA took part in the campaigns of the European Dyslexia Association 'Children at Risk of Dyslexia' and 'Early Recognition and Intervention'. It was very important because dyslexic children in our country are usually not diagnosed until the end of primary school (age 12), or at the end of *gymnasium* (age 15). It should, however, be done much earlier. In 1973 the learning of reading was introduced in the '0' grades – preparatory classes for 6-year-old children, which is actually still the kindergarten age – but 'the educational difficulties' may appear even before starting school. Therefore in the '0'-class it is already possible to recognize the symptoms of 'risk of dyslexia'.

Although the problem of early diagnosis of these difficulties has been known in Poland for a long time (Nartowska published books on this subject in 1980 and 1986), this knowledge did not function in practice. Even nowadays it happens in Poland that parents together with the pre-school teachers assume that a 6-year-old pupil is still a little child, therefore his or her difficulties are something quite natural at this age. They presume all the problems will solve themselves in the future as the child will 'grow out of it'.

The term 'children at risk of dyslexia' was popularized by Bogdanowicz in 1993 during the campaign of the PDA and the 11th All-Polish Conference on Early Prevention of Dyslexia. Since then it has been used in professional terminology and has caused the growth of society's awareness that prevention of dyslexia is necessary.

RECOGNITION

Theoretic assumptions determine the diagnostic procedure used to identify difficulties in reading and writing. Hence, the diagnostic examination includes evaluation at the level of the development of visual and auditory perception and memory, language functions, motor skills, sensorimotor integration, laterality and orientation in body and space schema. The starting point for the diagnosis of the potentially dyslexic child is the evaluation of intellectual efficiency using the Wechsler Intelligence Scale for Children (WISC-R). Quantity data as well as the profile of results are analysed in order to find the pattern specific for dyslexic children.

The next stage of formal assessment is diagnosing certain functions with a set of tests and trials, interview, observation and analysis of documents.

In order to assess the degree of developmental delay of diagnosed function the Indicator of Partial Developmental Deficit applied by Spionek is used (see the box below). The range of disturbances is estimated by the number of incorrectly developed functions which influence reading and writing.

$$\text{Indicator of Partial Developmental Deficit} = \frac{\text{delay of a given function}}{\text{chronological age}}$$

Interpretation of the Indicator:
Indicator above 0.20 – significant delay
Indicator above 0.30 – deep delay

Children should be fully diagnosed by an interdisciplinary team: psychologist, educator, speech therapist and sometimes a physician (e.g. neurologist, psychiatrist, optician) in order to receive remedial help best fitted to age, depth and range of disturbances.

REMEDIATION

In Poland the term 'educational therapy' is used to describe treatment through educational activities, the aim of which is to remove or reduce the developmental disturbances. This involves increasing the efficiency of disturbed functions and stimulation of undisturbed functions.

There are five levels of remedial help available for children with reading and writing difficulties:

- help of parents under teacher's guidance;
- remedial teaching in small so-called corrective-compensatory groups at schools;
- individual therapy in psychological-educational clinics (state or private);
- therapeutic classes (in primary schools and *gymnasium* only);
- day-care centres and wards providing intensive remedial teaching as well as medical therapy (few months stay).

Other possibilities of help include integration classes or schools, and therapeutic camps organized by the PDA.

Special educational services for children with dyslexia have been improving gradually in the past ten years, mainly thanks to the establishment of private therapeutic centres and to the activities of the PDA. Now our main goal is to develop the system of prevention of specific learning difficulties in reading and writing.

THE RIGHTS OF DYSLEXIC PUPILS IN POLISH SCHOOLS

In 1975 the Polish Ministry of Education published a leaflet considering qualifying children with developmental disturbances to appropriate forms of remedial teaching. The Act dating from 25th of May 1993 gave parents the possibility of asking the psychological-educational clinics for diagnosis and therapy, without referral from the school. It also enabled the provision of corrective-compensatory group activities for the children at risk of dyslexia in kindergartens and also created therapeutic classes in schools.

Since 1997 the Polish Dyslexia Association has been running a campaign providing equal educational chances for dyslexics. This problem was first addressed by the President of the PDA, Marta Bogdanowicz, in her presentation on 'The weaknesses and possibilities of people with special educational needs', during the conference of the Group for Family Matters which took place in the Polish Parliament on 17 May 1997 in Warsaw. The subject was then further discussed at the following conference on 'The Models of Care for Dyslexics in Poland' and published in some articles.

The next step of the campaign was addressing written appeals to the Ministry of Education and local educational authorities as well as institutions responsible for organizing the external examinations at the end of primary school. The same letters were also sent to the mass media (radio and TV). In our appeal we quoted the information on the rights of dyslexic children in other countries' school systems (see *International Book on Dyslexia*, ed. Salter and Smythe, 1997), the Warnock Report (1978), Articles 28 and 29 of the Convention on the Rights of the Child (United Nations, 1989) and the Act on the Educational System (of 7 September 1991).

The effect of this campaign was that some decrees of the Ministry of Education were published and also that the President of the Polish Dyslexia Association took part in the work of the Advisers Programme Board of the Central Examining Board (an institution subordinate to the Ministry of Education, but independent from the schools' and teachers' system of assessment of pupils).

New legislation of 15 January 2001 stated that parents have also the right to decide whether or not the child takes part in educational therapy as well as give permission to attend therapeutic classes and take the external exams in special conditions adapted to their special educational needs.

Dated 21 March 2001, the Decree of the Ministry of Education on Conditions and Ways of Grading, Classifying and Promoting the Students and Organizing the Examinations and Tests in Public Schools (*Legislation Journal*, 29/2001, p. 323) concerned the competence test conducted in the last grade of primary school, the *gymnasium* exam and the high school final exam (Baccalaureat – maturity exam) in the final grades.

It stated that:

> Pupils with dysfunctions have the right to be tested or examined in the form and conditions adjusted to their dysfunction, due to the opinion of public psychological-educational clinic or other public specialistic clinic. Such opinion should be dated from not later than 30th September in the year when the Test or Exam is conducted. (Chapter 4, Article 32.1)

A subgroup for Specific Learning Difficulties Pupils was established within the group for SEN Pupils of the Central Examining Board. It was the first time that dyslexic children had been recognized as part of the group for SEN Pupils. This subgroup in co-operation with the Regional Examining Board in Gdansk prepared the project on the conditions for external exams which take place in Poland from 2002 on the two levels of competence test and *gymnasium* exam. It was published as an Appendix to the Information Bulletin of Central Examining Board. The similar project for the 3rd level of exams – the Baccalaureat (the last class of high school) – the basis for entering the universities, was prepared by the Central Examining Board in co-operation with the subgroup mentioned above (published in Decree of the Ministry of Education and Sport, dated 7 January 2003, *Legislation Journal*, 26/2003, p. 225).

In another part of the Decree of the Ministry of Education dated 21 March 2001 concerning 'Assessing, classification and promoting pupils at schools for children and youths', the law was published which is basic to the internal school assessment:

> The teacher is obliged to adjust educational requirements mentioned in *Art. 4, p. 1* to the individual needs of a pupil with diagnosed learning difficulties (including specific learning difficulties) precluding realization of the requirements, according to the opinion of the psychological-educational clinic or other public specialist clinic. (Chapter 2, Article 6)

The Decree of the Ministry of Education and Sport, dated 24 April 2002 (*Legislation Journal*, 46/2002, p. 433) enabled certain non-public specialist clinics to give written opinions on dyslexia. It also gave the possibility of exempting children with severe dyslexia from learning a second foreign language at school (on parents' request).

Taking advantage of the rights

The conditions for diagnosing dyslexia are as follows:

- The child must have a written opinion (diagnosis) from public psychological-educational clinic or specialist clinic subordinate to the Ministry of Education or a PDA Clinic for Diagnosis and Therapy.
- The opinion must include a statement of occurrence of specific difficulties in reading and writing (developmental dyslexia).
- The opinion must be dated from not later than 30 September in the year in which the given examination is conducted.
- The opinion must be up to date and accepted by the parents of the child.

CONCLUSION

The rights of dyslexic children have been firmly established in Poland, thanks to the efforts of the PDA. Nevertheless, these rights are neither privileges, nor an excuse from work but give direction for systematic and adequate help according to the special educational needs of dyslexic children.

NOTE

1 This research was carried out by M. Bogdanowicz and A. Szalek.

REFERENCES

Bogdanowicz, M. (1978) Psychologiczna analiza trudności w pisaniu u dzieci. *Psychologia*, 1, 89–100.

Bogdanowicz, M. (1985a) Therapeutic care of children with reading and writing difficulties in Poland. In D.D. Duane and C.K. Leong, *Understanding Learning Disabilities: International and Multidisciplinary Views*. New York: Plenum Press.

Bogdanowicz, M. (1985b) Badania nad częstością występowania dysleksji, dysortografii i dysgrafii wśród polskich dzieci. *Psychologia*, 7, 143–156.

Bogdanowicz, M. (1993) Sensorimotor integration and special difficulties in acquiring skills. *Bulletin le Bon Départ*, 3, 1–18.

Bogdanowicz, M. (1996) The Good Start Method. *Bulletin le Bon Départ*, 1, 38–46.

Bogdanowicz, M. (1997) The awareness of dyslexia in Poland. In J. Waterfield (ed.), *Dyslexia in Higher Education: Learning along the Continuum*. Dartington Hall: University of Plymouth.

Bogdanowicz, M. (1999) Model kompleksowej pomocy osobom z dysleksją rozwojową – ocena stanu aktualnego i propozycje zmian w świetle reformy systemu edukacji. *Psychologia Wychowawcza*, 3, 217–227.

Bogdanowicz, M., Jaklewicz, H. and Loebl, W. (1969) Próba analizy specyficznych zaburzeń czytania i pisania. *Psychiatria Polska*, 3, 297–301.

Drath, A. (1959) Dysleksja. *Szkoła Specjalna* 4–5, 194–201.

Konorski, J. (1969) *Integracyjna działalność mózgu*. Warsaw: PWN.

Spionek, H. (1965) *Zaburzenia psychoruchowego rozwoju dziecka*. Warsaw: WsiP.

Spionek, H. (1973) *Zaburzenia w rozwoju uczniów a niepowodzenia szkolne*. Warsaw.

Tomaszewska, A. (2001) *Prawo do nauki dziecka z dysleksją rozwojową w świadomosci nauczycieli*. Kraków: Oficyta Wyd. Impuls.

Tomaszewski, T. (1963) *Wprowadzenie do psychologii*. Warsaw: PWN.

Zakrzewska, B. (1976) *Reedukacja dzieci z trudnościami w czytaniu i pisaniu*. Warsaw: WsiP.

ORGANIZATION

Polski Towarzystwo Dysleksji
Pomorska 68
80 343 Gdansk
Poland
Tel.: +48 58 5570531
Email: psymbg@univ.gda.pl

CHAPTER AUTHOR

Marta Bogdanowicz
Psychology Department
University of Gdansk
Gdansk
Poland
Email: Marta.bogdanowicz@wp.pl

DYSLEXIA IN RUSSIA

Tatiana Boldyreva and Olga B. Inshakova

UNDERSTANDING THE TERM DYSLEXIA IN RUSSIA

The term dyslexia, which is widely used in English-speaking countries, has a somewhat different meaning in Russia. It encompasses several disorders which are usually considered separately. The written language has two aspects – reading and writing. Reading and writing disorders are called dyslexia and dysgraphia, respectively.

Dyslexia is a partial reading disorder which is manifested in a slower rate of reading and in numerous specific errors. These errors are also of a persistent nature. Dysgraphia is a partial and specific writing disorder in which an inappropriate grapheme (letter) is chosen to designate the corresponding sound, or there is a syntactical disorder of written language. Such errors are of a fairly persistent nature.

This division is based principally on the fact that:

- dysgraphia is encountered two to three times more frequently than dyslexia;
- the degree of writing and reading difficulty can be different;
- there are descriptions of cases of 'pure' alexia without any serious writing disorder;
- there are cases of 'pure' agraphia without any reading disorder.

These last instances concern adults to a large extent. Agraphia and alexia in children can be the consequence of alalia or aphasia. The terms dyslexia and dysgraphia are used in Russia to designate reading and writing disorders resulting from the loss of speech (aphasia), and also resulting from under-development of the Higher Mental Functions (HMF, after A.R. Luria, the complex forms of conscious mental activity). Primary and secondary dyslexia and dysgraphia are differentiated. Primary reading and writing disorders are connected with aphasia and are caused by disorders in the upper cerebral cortex (in children and in adults).

Secondary reading and writing disorders in children are as a rule a combination of reading and writing disorders with spoken language problems, visual problems, optical spatial disorders, hearing disorders, etc.

International Book of Dyslexia: A Guide to Practice and Resources. Edited by Ian Smythe, John Everatt and Robin Salter. ISBN 0-471-49646-4. © 2004 John Wiley & Sons, Ltd.

Dyslexia and dysgraphia are often accompanied by dyslalia, mental retardation, rhino-alalia, dysartia, alalia and poor hearing, i.e. they appear in the structure of complex mental and speech disorders. They can manifest themselves independently in cases of left-hand-edness and bilingualism. The terms 'childhood dyslexia and dysgraphia' or 'evolutionary dyslexia and dysgraphia' are sometimes used for secondary dyslexia and dysgraphia.

As far as left-handed individuals are concerned, reading and writing disorders are very different in these cases. The disorders are more varied and, as a rule, do not correlate with the presence of speech disorders. The phenomenon of reversion (mirror-writing) is char-acteristically present in left-handed individuals.

The most serious and complex forms of dyslexia and dysgraphia are to be seen in cases of corrected left-handed individuals who now write with the right hand. Their mistakes are special and take the form of perception disorders and incorrect orthography of vowels (they cannot differentiate sounds by ear), and also soft consonants (reading and writing of letters). Vowel sounds are written and read incorrectly, even when stressed, where they are clearly audible.

Certain characteristic behaviour can be observed in this group of children which con-tributes to the development of dysgraphia and dyslexia. One kind of behaviour is *hyper-activity* (over-active) and the other is *hypoactivity* (under-active). Some 75 per cent of 'left-sided' persons are hyperactive, having difficulty with attention, low control level, etc., with the remaining 25 per cent being hypoactive, and having difficulties in switching on, attention (inhibition and irritation). Children can have great problems with their behav-iour such as studying and unwillingness to go to school. Sometimes the appearance of reading and writing difficulties of 'left-sided' children are the fault of the parents as they try to teach their children to do things (e.g. to write) with their right hand, which makes more problems for the left-handed child. 'Left-sided 'persons have left-side psycho-organization, which includes dominant left hand, leg, eye and ear. It is estimated that 10 per cent of children show reading and writing difficulties, of which only 4 per cent receive special help.

HELP FOR THE DYSLEXIC INDIVIDUAL

Logopaedists (speech and language therapists), defectologists and psychologists conduct special remedial work with parents of young children, trying to solve the problem of cor-rected left-handedness. Where this is inadequate, help can also come from the doctor. This reflects the multi-disciplinary approach to solving problems which is characteristic in Russia. The state gives support to parents and children suffering from dysgraphia and dyslexia in a national programme.

Remediation is carried out in special schools for children with serious speech problems including aphasia, cleft palate and stuttering, each of which can lead to reading and writing problems. There are six such schools in Moscow, as well as 400 ordinary schools where the help of speech therapists can be obtained.

THE TRAINING OF DYSLEXIA SPECIALISTS

The state trains specialists, who solve this problem in medical institutions (hospitals, polyclinics, sanatoria) and in establishments which are engaged in the education and upbringing of children (kindergartens, general education schools, special schools and boarding schools for children with serious speech problems). Specialist logopaedists are trained in special programmes in universities in faculties of correctional pedagogy. The curriculum consists of:

- direct professional training in the speciality of logopaedia: such subjects as logopaedia, psychology of speech, phonology, technology, etc., are studied in depth;
- special attention is given to medical subjects: neuropathology, psychophysiology, psychopathology, clinical mental retardation, etc;
- a large part of the curriculum is devoted to the study of psychology: general psychology, child and developmental psychology, pathopsychology, diagnostics, individual and group correctional work, etc.

In addition to this specialization of logopaedia, graduates also become practising psychologists. The second title gives the opportunity of doing remedial work on disorders in children's mental and social development, solving problems with behaviour and learning difficulties, and also doing work with parents. On completion of their studies graduates have a choice of becoming either a logopaedist or a psychologist. Whatever their choice, the knowledge which they have of a combined discipline helps in their work with speech problems of adults and children.

Special attention is paid to practical work which begins in the first year of their course. Students acquire the knowledge and skills to conduct logopaedic and psycho-pedagogical diagnoses, and also to use remedial methods to correct disorders.

HELP FOR DYSLEXIC CHILDREN

There are two degrees in the manifestation of writing and reading disorders in children:

- degree 1 – early evidence of dysgraphia and dyslexia in children aged 5–6 which is discovered at the time of the logopaedist's inspection at the children's polyclinic. This inspection is obligatory for all children before starting school. Special texts are used for this.
- degree 2 – all school-age children must undergo a compulsory inspection by the logopaedist during their first year at general education school.

Usually one logopaedist serves 25 primary classes (this could be one, two or three schools). After assessing the children the logopaedist selects those with dyslexia and dysgraphia and does correctional work with them using a special programme.

The work takes place two or three times a week for 45 minutes in the logopaedist's specially equipped room. Usually the remedial exercises continue for 1 to 1.5 years. The room could be situated in one of the schools. Exercises take place after normal lessons. The logopaedist decides the form of work for each child (group or individual). In the case of the writing or reading disorder arising during education in a second language, the exercises are conducted only individually. In our country a start has been made officially in developing such programmes. Older pupils can also be sent to the logopaedist's classroom. Among the logopaedist's duties is the education of teachers who have pupils in their classes who are working with the logopaedist, as well as doing special work with the parents.

In the case of serious problems in overcoming dyslexia and dysgraphia, special school conditions are needed where children stay for the entire school week (in special boarding schools for language disorders). If the dyslexia or dysgraphia is the result of aphasia in adults, then the patient first receives treatment for the restoration of spoken language, reading and writing while he or she is in hospital. The exercises are done with a logopaedist working in the department of speech therapy. The programme and quantity of lessons are individually selected. After leaving hospital, care of the patient is handed over to the logopaedist at the clinic near the patient's home. Exercises could take place at the patient's home if it is difficult for the patient to go out, or at the clinic. In the past two or three years private firms have developed which give treatment to overcome disorders of speech, reading and writing. Now parents and adults have the right to choose logopaedic, pedagogic and psychological treatment.

CHAPTER AUTHORS

Tatiana Boldyreva and Olga Inshakova
Special Education Department
Moscow State Education Pedagogical University
Moscow
Russia
Tel.: +7 095 214 0335
Email: olgainsh@land.ru

DYSLEXIA IN SCOTLAND

Elizabeth J. Reilly

INTRODUCTION

The education and legal systems in Scotland have always been different from those in England and have required separate legislation by the British Parliament in London. In June 1999 the Scottish Parliament was reconvened after a gap of almost 300 years and matters such as education and health are now wholly within the powers of our new Parliament. The new Scottish Executive, which is our equivalent of the government in London, is actively promoting policies designed to counter social exclusion and to promote life-long learning.

DYSLEXIA SCOTLAND

Dyslexia Scotland (formerly the Scottish Dyslexia Association) has 12 branches throughout Scotland, staffed mostly by volunteers, and a headquarters office in Stirling with a small number of paid staff who, among a myriad of other things, man a help-line five days a week. The work being done by volunteers and staff in Scotland is almost 'tailor-made' to assist the new Scottish Executive in promoting its policies. Dyslexia Scotland have responded to requests to comment on policy documents sent to us by the Executive, thus ensuring that we have a say in future policy, and we feel encouraged that we are being listened to.

To a large extent, although branches are involved in a variety of activities, holding meetings, conferences, etc., a great deal of their work is answering calls from parents who are desperate for help. In the majority of cases, parents report that they are at odds with their school trying to find out why their child is having difficulties.

Telephone calls to our head office help-line have increased by 400 per cent since 1999 to a staggering 6,300 calls in 2002. The staff who man the help-line have an extensive

International Book of Dyslexia: A Guide to Practice and Resources. Edited by Ian Smythe, John Everatt and Robin Salter. ISBN 0-471-49646-4. © 2004 John Wiley & Sons, Ltd.

knowledge of dyslexia. Callers include parents, adult dyslexics, teachers, lecturers, employers, doctors, nurses, speech therapists, occupational therapists, and recently more and more nurses working in psychiatric hospitals, etc.

Because of Scotland's geography, many of our outlying areas are sparsely populated and each year Dyslexia Scotland goes to such an area of the country to inform local people about dyslexia and instruct them in what is available in the way of information and help. Recently, our staff, together with Keda Cowling (author of *Toe by Toe*), had a very successful visit to the Western Isles.

EDUCATION POLICY

There is at the moment a lack of uniformity of educational policy or practice throughout the country. Based on feedback from our members, there are obvious areas of good practice and others of bad practice. Some local authorities appear to have no policy whatsoever regarding learning support for dyslexic children in the schools under their control and as an organization we are trying to influence change in these areas.

Legislation enacted many years ago introduced the concept of a Record of Needs (RON). Very briefly, this RON will contain a description of a child's special educational needs (SEN) and a statement as to how those needs will be met by the education authority concerned. Either of its own volition or at the request of the parents, the authority should carry out an assessment to determine a child's SEN and then decide whether a RON should be opened. Presuming that all who are involved in the assessment process agree with the description of the child's needs and the statement as to how the authority will meet these needs, then the parents will have a legally enforceable 'contract'.

Some education authorities will take the initiative to progress an assessment and prepare a fair and reasonable RON within a reasonable period of time. However, very often it is the parents who request an assessment which is carried out only after many months have passed and sometimes this results in a draft RON with which the parents strongly disagree. This often causes friction between the parents and the authority. Dyslexia Scotland's staff are able to inform parents of their rights in relation to applying for a RON and can help guide them through the process. Currently the Scottish Parliament are considering a new Draft Education Bill which will do away with the Record of Needs and hopefully legislate for something less cumbersome and more accessible to parents. We are involved in the consultation on these matters.

ADULT DYSLEXICS

There has been a sharp increase in the number of adult dyslexics contacting our help-line. I believe that this is partly because of Dyslexia Scotland raising awareness of dyslexia, but also because there has been more media coverage of the subject. A number of our branches now have adult groups attached to them.

In Scotland, Community Education Departments in local authorities have sections for Adult Basic Education (ABE), somewhere adults can go if they cannot read and write, and there they are given free tutoring, a second chance to learn. Dyslexia Scotland (DS) staff have given lectures to tutors in these departments so that the majority of the agency's tutors now have a working knowledge of dyslexia. DS, in partnership with ABE in a local authority, have recently developed a *Tutors Training Manual* to help tutors understand the most appropriate methods of assessing and teaching dyslexic adults. Work of this nature is continuing.

EFFECTS OF NON-DIAGNOSIS

Anyone who has knowledge of the reality of dyslexia will be familiar with the potential cascade effect of non-diagnosis or lack of remediation at an early age, e.g. truancy, disruptive behaviour in the classroom, violent and aggressive behaviour in late teens, or even criminal behaviour as an adult. Research carried out in a Scottish young offenders institution suggested that more than 50 per cent of the inmates are dyslexic to one degree or another. This figure is disturbing when looked at in relation to the percentage of the general population who suffer from dyslexia, i.e. 10 per cent. Our staff have been involved in giving lectures to prison tutors. In 2001, in partnership with the Education Adviser in the Scottish Prison Service, we developed a standardized screening and assessment process, together with a *Teachers Training Manual* to be used by all teachers working within the Scottish Prison Service.

CONCLUSION

There is no doubt that people in Scotland, both in the community at large, and in our education authorities in particular, are becoming more aware of dyslexia and the associated difficulties, and we are encouraged that many positive changes are taking place. However, there is still a great deal of work to be done.

ACKNOWLEDGEMENTS

Our work is possible because of the generosity of our funders: the Scottish Executive Life-Long Learning Department, the Dulverton Trust, the McRobert Trust, Lloyds TSB and the Gulbenkian Trust together with all the donations from individuals and companies. We are extremely grateful to them all.

ORGANIZATION

Dyslexia Scotland
Stirling Business Centre
Wellgreen
Stirling, FK8 2DZ
Scotland
Tel.: 01786 446650
Fax: 01786-471235
Email: info@dylsexia-in-scotland.org

CHAPTER AUTHOR

Elizabeth J. Reilly
Dyslexia Scotland
Stirling Business Centre
Wellgreen
Stirling. FK8 2DZ
Scotland

DYSLEXIA IN SINGAPORE

J.S. Daruwalla

THE DYSLEXIA ASSOCIATION OF SINGAPORE

The Dyslexia Association of Singapore (DAS) was started as a result of a Community Service Project of the Rotary Club of Raffles City, Singapore. A public forum on dyslexia was planned for April 1990. Speakers at this Forum included Marion Welchman, Jean Augur and Dr Lee Wei Ling, Consultant Paediatric Neurologist and Head of Learning Disorders Clinic at School Health Services. Dr Lee had made a study of 2,810 school children in 1990 and noted that the prevalence of dyslexia was 3.3 per cent. The Association was registered in 1991 and with the funds raised from a golf tournament organized by the Four Lions Clubs, our first teacher was employed. The stigma of having a learning difficulty was more or less removed when Mr Lee Kuan Yew, the former Prime Minister of Singapore, announced that he had mild dyslexia and donated a large sum of money to DAS. This created more public awareness, and there was a flood of inquiries.

In 2001, our Association celebrated its tenth anniversary. We have come a long way in our mission to serve the needs of dyslexic children in Singapore and increase public awareness of this learning difficulty.

Today, DAS provides remedial classes to nearly 400 primary and secondary dyslexic students in three learning centres. With the assistance of the Ministry of Education (MOE), dyslexic children in mainstream schools are being identified more quickly and referred to our Association for remedial help. An experienced and specially-trained teacher in each primary school, called the Learning Support Co-ordinator (LSC), helps to identify students who display signs and symptoms of dyslexia.

Increased professional sharing has helped to further strengthen the working relationship between DAS and MOE. LSCs and educational psychologists from MOE join our teachers in their training programmes. Our centre co-ordinators help to conduct yearly awareness talks to primary and secondary teachers as well as LSCs.

International Book of Dyslexia: A Guide to Practice and Resources. Edited by Ian Smythe, John Everatt and Robin Salter. ISBN 0-471-49646-4. © 2004 John Wiley & Sons, Ltd.

REMEDIAL CLASSES

Our Association conducts remedial classes twice a week for children outside their school hours at the three centres. Class size is kept to four students to maximize learning. All students who have been on the programme for at least six months are tested annually to review their progress. At the end of the academic year, parents are invited to a meeting with the class teacher to discuss the annual test results, their concerns and related issues. Annual parent-orientation sessions are held for parents of new students on the programme. This partnership between DAS and parents helps to ensure that students benefit more fully from attending the remedial classes.

MULTI-SENSORY TEACHING

We continue to place much emphasis on upgrading the skills of our teachers. Fellows from the Orton-Gillingham Academy of Practitioners and Educators regularly provide training in the multi-sensory approach to teaching dyslexic children. In-service workshops are held on related areas such as assessment and diagnosis, oral language difficulties, non-verbal learning difficulties and reading comprehension.

ASSESSMENT

The assessment arm of our Association has been expanded with more teachers helping to conduct screening. With increasing public awareness, more parents are coming forward on their own to have their children screened for dyslexia. We continue to receive referrals from other professionals in the medical and education fields.

FUNDING

Fund-raising is an annual affair for DAS which is a private, non-profit organization. Although MOE provides a per capita grant, our Association needs to raise funds annually to make up for the shortfall of S$600,000. DAS has been fortunate to receive generous donations from corporate sponsors and individuals. The money raised from fund-raising activities is used to provide more subsidies for students on the programme, to employ and train specialist staff and to purchase teaching and learning resources for the three centres.

DAS has made progress since its inception ten years ago. However, based on the conventional international estimate that 3 to 4 per cent of children in any population suffer from dyslexia, much more needs to be done to ensure that dyslexic children, who are part of Singapore's human resource, will receive the help that is needed to reach their full potential.

The direction for our Association in the next ten years is clear – how best to expand our services and meet the needs of more dyslexic children in Singapore.

As a first step, our Association held a Dyslexia Awareness Symposium in June 2002. This symposium reached out to parents and the public at large. Speakers included an educational psychologist who will be able to help in the assessment and diagnosis of dyslexia in a multi-lingual society.

We also envisage building a dyslexia-friendly school in either 2006 or 2007. This school will provide comprehensive primary school education for more severely dyslexic children as well as remedial classes to help the less severely dyslexic children cope with their literacy difficulties.

Another core focus area includes working with the MOE on policies affecting dyslexic children. Dyslexic students currently receive accommodations such as extra time for tests and examinations as well as exemption from learning a second language on a case-by-case basis. More concessions can be given to level the playing field for dyslexic students in the mainstream schools.

Our Association must also encourage and initiate local research on dyslexia in Singapore. The Singapore situation is unique because it is a melting pot of languages. Available international literature on dyslexia and multi-lingualism tends to focus on research done on difficulties with the Chinese script. We have dyslexics who have difficulties with Malay and the Indian languages. Local research will help us ultimately to better understand the needs of dyslexics in Singapore. Only then will we be able to achieve the best practice in remedial teaching. It will be a great challenge for our Association to achieve the goals set. However, we must remember: 'Not everything that is faced can be changed; but nothing can be changed until it is faced' (Anonymous).

ORGANIZATIONS

Dyslexia Association of Singapore
Fengshan Primary School
307 Bedok North Road
Singapore 469680
Tel.: 65 64445700
Fax: 65 64447900
Website: www.das.org.sg
Email: leesiang_das@org.sg

CHAPTER AUTHOR

J.S. Daruwalla
President
Dyslexia Association of Singapore
c/o Daruwalla Orthopaedic Spine and Hand Surgery Pte Ltd
3 Mount Elizabeth #03-01/06
Mount Elizabeth Medical Centre
Singapore 228510
Email: jimmyd@singnet.com.sg

DYSLEXIA IN SOUTH AFRICA

Catherine Hattingh

INTRODUCTION

The total population of South Africa in 2002 is estimated at 45 million people. The population is made up of various races that represent at least 24 languages and numerous dialects. According to information supplied by the Education Department, 7,527,895 primary learners attended 16,863 primary schools and 4,072,470 secondary learners attended 5,624 secondary schools in 2000. In 2000 27,021 learners attended special schools or special learning centres. The total number of learners in South Africa in 2000 was estimated at 11,903,455 (Education Department: Census 2000).

LANGUAGES

The interim Constitution of the Government of National Unity granted equal status to 11 languages, i.e. Afrikaans, English, Pedi, Xhosa, Zulu, Sotho, Tsonga, Venda, Tswana, Ndebele and Swazi. Up to 1994 South Africa was a bilingual country with only Afrikaans and English as official languages. Less than 10 per cent of the South African population are native English speakers, but show a clear preference for English as the medium of instruction because all the main universities, technikons and technical colleges still present their courses in English or Afrikaans. Proficiency in English is therefore seen as a means to certain opportunities in further education and allows people to improve their social status, privileges and power.

At present the school system for black schoolchildren is an English-medium system from the commencement of the fifth year of schooling. Most of the time they transfer from mother tongue instruction to English before they have gained adequate grounding in their mother tongue and before they have sufficient vocabulary in English. Failure to reach adequate levels of language skills in the mother tongue before the introduction of English means that many children suffer the negative effect of semi-lingualism.

International Book of Dyslexia: A Guide to Practice and Resources. Edited by Ian Smythe, John Everatt and Robin Salter. ISBN 0-471-49646-4. © 2004 John Wiley & Sons, Ltd.

South African native languages also differ hugely from the Germanic languages of English and Afrikaans. For example, all words in South African native languages end in vowels, while many words in English end in consonants – this fact causes many pronunciation mistakes, leading to reading and spelling mistakes. Sometimes teachers are not properly trained and are not aware of the background or language tracks of these children. Such a child can easily be labelled as dyslexic or slow.

Most of the South African native languages as well as Afrikaans have 'shallow orthographies', i.e. the spelling–sound correspondence is direct. Given the rules, anyone can immediately read the words correctly.

English, however, is regarded as having a 'deep', irregular orthography – indicating a complex correspondence between spelling and pronunciation which causes black schoolchildren (and white Afrikaans schoolchildren) to experience difficulties in reading and spelling in English.

Most vernacular languages in South Africa have been taught as subjects but left as a medium of instruction until they reach scientific capability. This placed a serious stranglehold on the cultural development of indigenous vernaculars, and constitutes a serious setback to the cultural consciousness of learners (Kunutu, in Engelbrecht *et al.*, 1996, p. 269).

LEGISLATION AND POLICIES IN EDUCATION

The development of specialized education in South Africa is different from other countries because of the philosophical and political influences over many decades. Up to 1994 separated, segregated and differentiated education was implemented for the various ethnic groups (White, Coloured, Black, Asian) by the central government. Special education was only available for white school learners. Special schools were developed for (white) deaf, blind, epileptic, cerebral palsied and physically disabled children, children with minimal brain dysfunction, autistic and severely handicapped children. Specialized education for disabled children from other population groups developed much more slowly, leading to severe discrepancies in both quality and quantity of such provision (du Toit, in Engelbrecht *et al.*, 1996, p. 11).

Since the first democratic elections for all South African citizens in April 1994 a huge effort has been made to redress these imbalances. In February 1995 with the publication of the *White Paper on Education and Training in a Democratic South Africa: First Steps to Develop a New System*, the following objectives were set for reconstruction:

- basic right to education, irrespective of race, class, gender, creed, or age;
- life-long education and training of good quality;
- open access to education;
- redressing of educational inequalities;
- a unitary education system;
- total development of all learners.

Services for special educational needs are at present governed and partially administered at national level, but there is autonomy at the provincial, district and school levels. In terms of the reorganization of the Department of Education, 'Remedial Education' falls under the Directorate for Special Needs in each of the country's nine provinces. The Directorates have two arms: a special education arm which looks at specialized schools; and a learning support arm which aims to develop learning support in the mainstream. The Education Department is looking for ways to redistribute large resources to make them available to all the children in South Africa.

OUTCOMES-BASED EDUCATION

At present the outcomes-based education (OBE) is followed throughout all the provinces in South Africa as directed by the Education Department. The outcomes-based education system is Intended to ensure that all pupils are able to achieve to their maximum ability and are equipped for lifelong learning. It is a learner-centred process where the learning process is considered as important as what is learnt. Teachers are facilitators and learners are encouraged to explore and discover new learning concepts for themselves. This system has had mixed results because of various factors such as inadequate teacher training, overcrowded classrooms, poor resources, etc. Compulsory education is up to 15 years or Grade 9. Until 1994 there was no free or compulsory education for African learners. Primary education starts in the year that the learner turns 7 and lasts for 7 years (Grades 1–7).

In order to attend a South African university, a secondary school learner must graduate from secondary school, which is a 12-year programme. A Matriculation Exemption is required. The learner must have taken tour or more subjects from the following groups for a minimum of three years: English, a second language (usually Afrikaans), Mathematics, Natural Sciences (Biology and/or Science), Accounting, Music, Biblical Studies, or Technical Drawing. The learner must take a minimum of six subjects, four of which must be on the higher grade (which must include English, and a second language) with the possibility of taking a 7th, 8th or 9th subject, which would add to their grade point average if passed.

South African Technikons are recognized tertiary-level institutions. Technikons provide career-orientated programmes, which combine theoretica and experiential learning.

DEFINITION AND TERMINOLOGY

Normally a distinction is made between general and specific learning disabilities. General learning disabilities also include specific learning disabilities. The following can be regarded as factors that can cause general learning disabilities:

- intellectual retardation;
- physical and sensory malfunction;
- illnesses;
- environmental influences and poor stimulation during early childhood years;
- emotional disturbances (trauma);
- specific learning disabilities (brain dysfunction and developmental dysfunction).

In the case of South Africa, 40–50 per cent of black school learners fall into the category of learning disabled due to the above mentioned factors which are mainly due to sociopolitical ideologies in South Africa over many years.

Learners with specific learning disabilities are those children who fail to achieve their full intellectual and academic potential despite adequate and quality education, normal sensory development, cultural background, emotional stability and motivation. Ross (in

Behr, 1988, p 167) also gave the following definition for learning disability: 'A learning disabled child is a child of at least average intelligence whose academic performance is impaired by a developmental lag in the ability to sustain selective attention.'

Dyslexia, regarded as a specific learning disability in South Africa, is, however, a concept not widely used or addressed, because of the huge number of reading disabilities found in learners because of other factors that are not of neurological or psychological origin. Ogilvy (1994, p. 60) even questioned the usefulness of the classification of dyslexia as a specific learning disability in South Africa saying that 'a separate diagnostic category cannot be justified to describe a condition which is neither distinct in terms of aetiology or presenting symptoms or in terms of what you do about it'. Kriegler (1989) pointed out that, even if such a category does indeed exist, it is hardly relevant in the current context of South African education, fraught as it is with so many more obvious sources of learning difficulties.

It is felt that if the problems that cause general learning disabilities can be eliminated and proper remedial intervention takes place, it will redress the present situation in South Africa to a large extent.

Illiteracy is a major problem in South Africa and it is estimated that up to 70 per cent of the rural population in some areas suffer from it (Wilson and Ramphele, 1989). Illiteracy is mainly due to environmental disadvantages. Children who suffer from reading disabilities usually have parents who are illiterate. These children were not exposed to a rich language environment and did not come into contact with print until they attended school. Children from illiterate communities, however, do not fit the label dyslexia.

IDENTIFICATION AND ASSESSMENT

Psychologists in school clinics as well as in private practices use a variety of assessment instruments – ranging from locally developed to standardized tests such as the Wechsler tests. Many of the tests are not standardized for the South African population and virtually no adaptive and intelligence tests exist or have been developed for and standardized to Africans.

In 1980 a cognitive research unit was established at the University of the Witwatersrand in Johannesburg. This led to the development of the Literacy Assessment Battery (LAB) to evaluate children in the Soweto area near Johannesburg who attended the school guidance clinic at the Chris Hani Baragwanath Hospital. At present the battery exists in three languages: English, Afrikaans and Pedi. It consists of six assessments, each containing a series of tests of orthographic, phonological, semantic, syntactic and morphological knowledge, and spelling. Although each test is designed for first language usage, the battery is flexible. The same tests can be used in one language alone, to provide a deeper understanding of the disorder, or comparisons can be made between languages, making the battery suitable for bilinguals or multilinguals.

Developmental norms have been collected for all the tests and for the different languages, making it possible to compare the performance of the poor reader or speller with a peer group of normal readers or spellers (Engelbrecht *et al.*, 1996, p. 364).

Much still needs to be done in terms of standardizing tests for school learners in order to identify learners with reading disabilities in primary and secondary schools. In the case of dyslexia, standardized reading and spelling tests are used (where available) to diagnose the extent of the reading disability. An individual remedial programme is then developed and implemented by private remedial teachers.

INTERVENTION AND RESOURCES

Vigorous attempts are made to redress the imbalances in education. University departments of special education and other organizations, such as the South African Association for Learning Disabilities (SAALED), have contributed research and produced publications directed at influencing policy at the national, regional and local levels. The greatest concern has been with the large number of learners who fall into the category of learning disabled due to factors such as environmental deprivation. The logical action at the moment is to mainstream learners with special needs while the process of redistributing services, resources and personnel to all learners and schools should take place as soon as possible.

There is at present a move away from the individualistic-medical approach to a more systemic-preventative approach in special education. Services are aimed to be predominantly preventative, dealing with environmental stresses. Emphasis is placed on the development of an optimal teaching and learning environment for all (NEPI, 1992). Mainstreaming of learners with special educational needs is the long-term goal.

The role of the remedial teachers is changing in order to serve a greater number of schools and act as a teacher support rather than work directly with the learners. Few black remedial teachers have been trained properly in the past, but that situation is also changing.

TEACHER TRAINING

Up to 1993 and the National Education Policy Investigation into Special Education (NEPI), educational specialists worked in isolation, without consultation with the National Government. In 1994 the Committee for Teacher Education Policy (COTEP) published *Norms and Standards: Governance Structures for Teacher Education* with the fundamental aim to 'teach effectively in order to facilitate learning'. After 1994 it was agreed that all teachers must receive training in basic special education. To qualify them for specialized education a Further Diploma in Education (Special Education Needs) is required. Such courses are presented at some universities in South Africa and teacher training colleges.

ADVOCACY GROUPS

The South African Association for Learning and Educational Difficulties (SAALED) focuses on all learners with special educational needs, whether it is a dysfunction in the learner, a disabling environment or the interaction between the two.

THE REMEDIAL FOUNDATION

The Remedial Foundation of South Africa is developing and promoting remedial education in South Africa with special emphasis on the 'educationally challenged' communities. In 1995 it launched a National Equal Education Directory Services (NEEDS) to provide telephone counselling and information to parents and teachers.

EXAMINATION AND CURRICULUM PROVISIONS

After psychological and educational assessments have been made, extra time can be allowed in examinations, or in severe cases of dyslexia they can be conducted orally.

Adult Basic Educational Training (ABET) centres focus on basic literacy and numeracy in adults. These centres are available throughout South Africa.

THE WAY AHEAD

The most urgent educational need in South Africa today is for special educational support in the acquisition of basic educational skills which have been delayed or denied to approximately 75,000 learners through lack of access to, or the inadequacy of, the existing educational system.

REFERENCES

Behr, A.L. (1988) Toward a megatheory of learning disabilities. *Journal of Learning Disabilities,* 21(4), 230–232.

Committee for Teacher Education Policy (1994) *Norms and Standards: Governance Structures for Teacher Education.* Cape Town: COTEP.

Education Department: Census 2000.

Engelbrecht, P., Kriegler, S.M. and Booysen, M.I. (1996) *Perspectives on Learning Disabilities.* Pretoria: J.L. van Schaik.

Kriegler, S. (1989) The learning disabilities paradigm: Is it relevant in the South African context? *SAALED Conference Proceedings.* Pretoria: University of Pretoria.

National Education Policy Investigation (NEPI) (1992) *Support Services.* Johannesburg: NEPI.

Ogilvy, C.M. (1994) What is the diagnostic significance of specific learning disabilities? *School Psychology International,* 15(1), 55–68.

South Africa, Dept. of Education (1995) *White Paper on Education and Training in a Democratic South Africa.* Pretoria: Government Printer.

Wilson, F. and Ramphele, M. (1989) *Uprooting Poverty: The South African Challenge.* Cape Town: David Philip.

ORGANIZATIONS

SAALED
PO Box 2404
Cape Town 7740
South Africa

The Remedial Foundation
PO Box 32207
Braamfontein 2017
Johannesburg
South Africa

CHAPTER AUTHOR

Catherine Hattingh
The University of the Free State
PO Box 339
Bloemfontein 9300
South Africa
Email: Hattcm@rd.uovs.ac.za

DYSLEXIA IN SWEDEN

Bodil Andersson

INTRODUCTION

Sweden today has about 9 million inhabitants. Every fifth person in Sweden is either an immigrant or has at least one parent who was born outside Sweden. The major immigrant languages spoken are Finnish, Arabic, Persian, Serbian and Spanish. Following a new law (April 2000), the country now has five official minority languages which entitles speakers of Sami, Finnish, Meänkieli (Tornedalen Finnish), Yiddish or Romany in certain regions to receive parts of societal information in their native language. A parliamentary commission has been appointed to investigate whether the majority language, Swedish, should also receive official status.

Sweden has a long history of reading instruction, originally for religious reasons: everybody should learn to read the word of God in the Bible. At the turn of the seventeenth century, Sweden was virtually a country of readers. Even then, literacy demands were high and an illiterate person was in fact not allowed to marry.

Internationally, Sweden has always held one of the top positions in reading ability. This has been confirmed by a number of reading studies such as the SIALS/OECD report (2000). The most recent example is the result from the PISA study, where 15-year-olds in 31 countries were compared for skills in reading, reading comprehension, applied maths and science. However, societal demands on literacy skills are extremely high in Sweden, which is a crucial aspect of reading/writing difficulties. In the Swedish labour market, hardly any manual jobs exist any longer. There is an increasing number of people whose literacy skills are inadequate in relation to society's literacy pressure. As many as 25 per cent of the Swedish population are said to suffer from this type of 'functional reading/writing problem'. The concern expressed by politicians and expert teachers about the literacy situation in society seems appropriate.

International Book of Dyslexia: A Guide to Practice and Resources. Edited by Ian Smythe, John Everatt and Robin Salter. ISBN 0-471-49646-4. © 2004 John Wiley & Sons, Ltd.

PREVALENCE OF DYSLEXIA

The prevalence of dyslexia in Sweden is estimated at about 5 per cent by almost all organizations in the Swedish reading field. However, definitional issues are much debated at present and many people call for discussion beyond the level of a sharply marked-off concept of dyslexia, as reading and writing difficulties are moving targets and the purpose of an assessment must always be to take proper action in a unique situation. Adopting the terminology of the World Health Organization (WHO), handicap occurs only when a person with a disability confronts a non-adapted environment. In other words, the gap between the societal demands on reading and writing skills and the nature of a reading/writing disabled person's disability will determine the level of handicap. This is captured by modern handicap politics in Sweden, including dyslexia.

The view on dyslexia has shifted with political trends over the years. During the 1970s, reading problems were mainly regarded as a social problem. Struggling readers were said to constitute an extended lower end of the normal distribution curve and hence dyslexia 'did not exist'.

THE FMLS

To give the people affected a voice in Swedish society, the main user organization for people with reading and writing difficulties, the FMLS, was formed in 1979. The FMLS grew stronger during the 1980s and was recognized as a handicap organization in 1990 by a governmental council, which meant the FMLS became a body to which the government can send proposals for consideration. Many people have interpreted this as the acknowledgement of the concept of dyslexia and it being officially agreed upon, but this is not quite the case.

In the 1980s, the dominant belief about reading difficulties was that it was a matter of maturity, obviously inconsistent with an interest in assessment and diagnosis. Many students and worried parents were reassured they should 'wait and see'. During this time, a state of conflict developed between reading teachers who applied a whole word method, and those in favour of a phonics approach. In 1989, the Swedish Dyslexia Association was formed to bring together professionals in the reading field.

MAJOR CHANGES IN POLICY

The 1990s saw major changes in Sweden. Several efforts during the Literacy Year of 1990, as proclaimed by the UN, increased understanding for the reading disabled in Sweden. A successful nation-wide campaign was arranged in 1997 to raise the public's awareness about dyslexia/reading and writing problems, directed by the FMLS and the Swedish Dyslexia Association and others. Many dyslexia resource centres started in the 1990s, along with teacher training courses and courses for psychologists and speech and language therapists. A large number of conferences have also been arranged.

Having reading and writing difficulties in the fast-moving information society can lead to far-reaching consequences. There is a slight over-representation of people with reading and writing problems among the unemployed in Sweden. In 1998, the Swedish National

Labour Market Administration therefore appointed the County Labour Board of Stadshagen, Stockholm, a national resource centre for competence regarding reading and writing difficulties and unemployment issues.

However, the 1990s was a time of financial stringency and as a consequence, many schools had to cut their resources for students with special needs. The number of special education teachers was reduced and reading disabled students received less help. Inclusion became the term of justification, but this was in many ways a false expression as inclusion was negatively caused by the stretched economy. Quite logically, in 1992 an organization for parents of dyslexic children was founded. This organization, called the FDB, supports families, improves the co-operation between homes and schools and strives towards early intervention.

Most Swedish children attend pre-school. The link between early phonemic awareness and later reading ability is well known through, for example, the Bornholm project (1988). Activities to enhance the prerequisites for reading and writing are being practised in most pre-schools.

SWEDISH SCHOOLS AND REMEDIATION

Until recently, the age of school entrance has been seven. Now, there is an integration between the last year of pre-school and the first formal school year and children may start formal schooling at the age of 6. Swedish schools were state-governed until the late 1980s, when local government replaced that system. There is now an increasing number of private schools, which was almost unheard of ten years ago.

The type, level and volume of intervention for reading disabled students vary with local conditions. There used to be a supplementary course programme of 6 months to 1.5 years for classroom teachers to become remediation teachers whose task was to work with children hands-on. However, for the past ten years, remediation teachers have no longer been specially trained. Instead there is a 1.5-year programme for teachers who wish to become special education teachers. Special education teachers may specialize in differents strands but not all become skilled in literacy issues. Supervision is an important part of their job, as the idea is to have the special education teachers supervise the ordinary classroom teachers. Some spend all their time supervising, others less, but the consequences of this change are obvious: fewer reading disabled children meet specialists face to face.

The current remediation debate in Swedish schools focuses on whether remediation should take place on a one-to-one basis or within the classroom. Some claim it is stigmatizing for a student to leave the classroom for training and think little of such intervention. Others say individual remediation, or in a small group, is crucial.

Around 70 per cent of Swedes have completed a comprehensive upper secondary education of three years or have a university degree, compared to about 45 per cent on average within the OECD. However, around 20 per cent of the upper secondary school students do not pass in the core subjects of Swedish, English and Mathematics and are therefore excluded from university level studies. Among students with an immigrant background, the figure is a depressing 40 per cent.

According to the view of the FMLS, there should be no need for special schools for dyslexic students. Instead, ordinary schools should be forced to learn to adapt their teaching methods and, of course, receive enough money to support the special needs of the students. This philosophy is in line with the message of the 1994 Salamanca Declaration by UNESCO, which clearly states that special educational efforts should aim at non-segregational goals.

A CONSENSUS PROJECT

As previously mentioned, many dyslexia-oriented courses for teachers started during the 1990s, representing a variety of theoretical approaches to dyslexia. The National Agency for Education initiated a nation-wide consensus project run by Professor Mats Myrberg, addressing the intervention methods used with dyslexic children as well as definitional issues, interviewing skilled teachers and researchers representing different disciplines. This project will finish in 2003.

Sadly, although the majority of active researchers basically agree on the definition of dyslexia, there is still much confusion out in the field, often to the detriment of the person in need of help. Many professional groups are involved – special education teachers, psychologists, medical doctors, speech and language therapists – and there is no official, overall agreed-upon definition or 'cut-off point' which all groups accept. Different professionals use different tests and they do not always understand each other's technical terminology. The term 'dyslexia' is used by some as an umbrella term for various symptoms such as poor, slow decoding and bad spelling; others use it to describe a condition that is thought to be the *cause* of those typical overt symptoms.

ASSESSMENT

There is no Swedish legislation concerning the right to make a diagnosis. According to the National Board of Health and Welfare (2000), it is

> customary within the health service to have a registered medical doctor or a registered psychologist carrying out the assessment, but anyone with sufficient skills can do it. An assessment requires pedagogical competence as well as qualifications from the health system.

This leaves a lot to interpretation and covers only the custom in the health system. Within the unemployment services, it is normally a psychologist who does the assessment; in hospitals it is usually a speech and language therapist. In schools, there is a variety of solutions, with practice varying with local conditions. The prevailing situation is to have either a trained special education teacher or a school psychologist carrying out the assessment. In general, teachers avoid the word 'diagnosis' as it belongs in a medical paradigm, rather than a pedagogical one. Most teachers tend to use the term 'reading and writing difficulties', as that is what is obvious in the teaching situation. Sometimes, the reading disabled pupil is referred to a speech and language therapist at the hospital for an assessment (in Sweden, it is still very unusual for speech and language therapists to be employed by schools). Some schools practise a method of team assessment, for example, by co-ordinating the evaluations by a medical doctor, a special education teacher and a psychologist. Many professionals believe a team assessment is the way forward, realizing the complex and multidimensional nature of reading problems.

For diagnosis, many medical doctors and psychologists rely on the DSM-IV. A few are advocates of the so-called discrepancy criterion, which means dyslexia is defined as a discrepancy between IQ and reading achievement, despite a lack of poor criteria. However, most Swedish researchers and practitioners have now acknowledged the limited use of the discrepancy criterion, as convincingly proved by researchers such as Siegel (1989) and Berninger (2001). Adopting the discrepancy criterion means accepting a 'wait to fail' attitude, because the desired discrepancy cannot be securely obtained until a child is 9–10 years of age. The majority would reason in accordance with a definition focusing on congenital word-decoding difficulties and a core phonological deficit, as presented by Høien and Lundberg (2000). However, recent findings from dyslexia studies in other papers by researchers such as Smythe and Everatt (2000) along with reports by Wolf *et al.* (2000) and others on the impact of fluency and visual factors in Swedish have created a desire for some amendments.

Many people in the reading field would welcome more consistency in assessment procedures, but perhaps equally important is improving the ways the implication of assessment findings are put into practice. At present, schools are obliged by the law to produce individual educational plans for students with 'special needs'. In many schools, this works well, but there are substantial problems associated with such vague wording as 'special needs' when it comes to reading/writing issues. In the light of the history of the Swedish reading debate, it sometimes means the student's problems are waved aside. Who decides whether 'special needs' exist? Whose assessment is valid? Clarification is needed. There is also a gap between the student's rights and the economic reality: money is often lacking to fulfil what the law claims.

ASSISTIVE TECHNOLOGY

The problem emerges also in issues regarding assistive technology. Today, it is difficult for a Swedish schoolchild to get a computer with appropriate software to facilitate reading and writing for the above reasons concerning the diagnosis. Strangely though, at university level it is a lot easier. The National Agency for Higher Education has created a list of people trusted to make high-quality assessments, and if the student is judged to have dyslexia by such a person, they are allowed to undergo the Swedish Scholastic Assessment Test (an admission test used for selection to higher education) using 50 per cent longer time. Once a dyslexic student has managed to get into university and is registered by a handicap coordinator, there is normally extensive help available (prolonged time in examinations, talking books, computer technology, etc.). The Swedish universities register the number of students with a disability. In 1990, there was one disabled student in 700 whole-year students; in 2000, this number had changed to 1 out of 120. The majority of the registered disabled students today are dyslexics. The Insurance Office often supports reading disabled people in working life who need assistive technology; at other times the employer will pay the expenses, but practice and level of support vary.

Another side to the matter is the question of accessible teaching aids. There has been a conflict between the need for adapted material for disabled persons (ebooks, talking books, etc.) and the copyright issues with the authors and publishers, in reality making it impossible to produce the material needed. This is currently being looked into by the government.

FUTURE AREAS OF INTEREST

In the future, there are some areas that deserve particular attention. Apart from the consensus discussions, multilingualism is also an issue along with compensation techniques.

The multilingualism issue

Swedish students do well in literacy compared to their peers in many countries; however, there is also a reverse to this coin: the literacy achievement of students with an immigrant background. From an international perspective, Sweden is not doing well in this field. There is a growing interest in ways to identify specific reading and writing difficulties and develop teaching methods among people whose first language is not Swedish. A project with Spanish-speaking dyslexics was recently carried out in Stockholm by SIOS, the Co-operation Group for Ethnic Associations in Sweden (www.sios.org/siosengelsk.htm). The project raised important questions concerning identification and intervention.

Compensation techniques

Dr Christer Jacobson of Växjö University carried out a follow-up study of a group of reading disabled 8-year-olds and found that seven years later, they were still behind their peers in reading development. Furthermore, Jacobson (1999) showed that these students receive lower grades in all subjects although controlled for general intelligence and aptitude. These findings reinforce the need for compensation techniques – in the spirit of WHO, to bridge the gap between the reading disability and the literacy demands, thus reducing the level of handicap.

The ICT Commission was set up by the Swedish government as the Advisory Board in the field of Information Technology. On behalf of the ICT Commission, Torbjörn Lundgren – an author and himself a dyslexic – has written a report on the ICT needs in the dyslexia field, which is hoped to have a major impact on the development in the coming years (Lundgren, 2001).

REFERENCES

Berninger, V. (2001) Understanding the 'lexia' in dyslexia: A multidisciplinary team approach to learning disabilities. *Annals of Dyslexia*, 51. Baltimore, MD: The International Dyslexia Association.

Høien, T. and Lundberg, I. (2000) *Dyslexia: From Theory to Practice*. Dordrecht: Kluwer Academic Publishers.

Jacobson, C. (1999) How persistent is reading disability? Individual growth curves in reading. *Dyslexia*, 5, 78–93.

Lundgren, T. (2001) *IT-satsningar på området läs- och skrivsvårigheter/dyslexi.* [IT efforts in the field of reading and writing difficulties/dyslexia.] Report written for the ICT Commission. Rapport 42/2001. Stockholm: IT-kommissionen.

The National Board of Health and Welfare (2000) *Diagnos av specifika inlärningssvårigheter/dyslexi.* Dnr 52-3377/2000 (response to enquiry from Uppsala University).

Siegel, L. (1989) Why we do not need intelligence scores in the definition and analysis of learning disabilities. *Journal of Learning Disabilities*, 22, 512–518.

Smythe, I. and Everatt, J. (2000) Dyslexia diagnosis in different languages. In L. Peer and G. Reid (eds), *Multilingualism, Literacy and Dyslexia*. London: David Fulton Publishers.

Wolf, M., Bowers, P. and Biddle, K. (2000) Naming-speed processes, timing and reading: A conceptual review. *Journal of Learning Disabilities*, 33, 387–407.

ORGANIZATIONS

Förbundet FMLS
(The Swedish Association for Persons with Difficulties in Reading and Writing/Dyslexia)
Brahegatan 20
SE-114 37 Stockholm
Sweden
Tel.: +46 8 665 17 00
Email: info@fmls.nu
Website: www.fmls.nu

Svenska Dyslexiföreningen
(The Swedish Dyslexia Association)
Karolinska Institutet
Retzius väg 8
SE-171 77 Stockholm
Sweden
Tel.: +46 8 728 6825
Email: svenska.dyslexiforeningen@neuro.ki.se
Website: www.ki.se/dyslexi

Föräldraföreningen för Dyslektiska Barn (FDB)
(The Association for Parents of Dyslexic Children)
Surbruunsg 42 1 tr, ö.g.
S-113 48 Stockholm
Sweden
Tel.: +46 8 612 06 56
Email: dyslexi@fdb.nu
Website: www.fdb.nu (Swedish only)

CHAPTER AUTHOR

Bodil Andersson
Åldermansgatan 5B, 2 tr.
SE-227 36 Lund
Sweden
Tel.: +46 702 71 0033
Email: bodil.andersson@bredband.net

DYSLEXIA IN SWITZERLAND

Susanne Bertschinger

INTRODUCTION

There is a special cultural framework in Switzerland. Most people know that Switzerland is a quadrilingual country although the official languages are Swiss German (approximately 74 per cent), French (approximately 20 per cent), Italian (approximately 5 per cent) and Romansch (approximately 1 per cent).

Over and above the 'normal' problems associated with dyslexia, Switzerland has the added difficulty of having to integrate the different information and therapy systems of four languages. Furthermore, each of the 12 Cantons into which the country is divided has its own independence in matters of education and culture; it is not even possible for the same language areas to be associated together.

SPEECH THERAPY CENTRES

In Switzerland, kindergarten teachers are often not well enough informed about the different types of problems and difficulties experienced by the dyslexic child. The local Speech Therapy Centre would be the best contact point for parents or kindergarten and secondary school teachers if they are concerned about the progress of their children in school. The centres are important points of contact although not all children with difficulties are dyslexic. This may only be established by an assessment of the child's difficulties.

The centres can suggest the possibility of spreading the first class over two years or suggesting speech therapy to assist in catching up with linguistic problems, or even suggesting psychomotoric therapy to assist in the improvement in writing, body and general awareness.

International Book of Dyslexia: A Guide to Practice and Resources. Edited by Ian Smythe, John Everatt and Robin Salter. ISBN 0-471-49646-4. © 2004 John Wiley & Sons, Ltd.

PSYCHOLOGICAL SERVICE CENTRES

There are also Psychological Service Centres which are responsible for assessing learning or behaviour. The centres may also decide whether or not therapy is necessary. If therapy is necessary, the responsible school authority has to assume the costs, therefore these services are in a very important position. At the present time, children who live in the larger cities have to wait for approximately six months for an examination of their problems, so much valuable time is lost.

If dyslexic children are to receive the help that they definitely will need in overcoming their difficulties (and therefore having a chance of reaching their potential in life), it is imperative that their problems are recognized at an early stage (i.e. preferably in kindergarten), identified as being those associated with dyslexia and then given the support at school of the appropriate teaching for their specific difficulties. This means, of course that teacher training of teachers is vital and that the staff at the Speech Therapy and Psychological Service Centres have to be given some understanding of dyslexia.

ORGANIZATION

Verband Dyslexie Schweiz
Alpenblick 17
8311 Brütten
Switzerland
Tel.: +41 52 345 04 61
Email: sekretariat@verband-dyslexie.ch

CHAPTER AUTHOR

Susanne Bertschinger
Verband Dyslexie Schweiz
Alpenblick 17
8311 Brütten
Switzerland
Email: sekretariat@verband-dyslexie.ch

DYSLEXIA IN TAIWAN

Wei-Pai Blanche Lue

TERMINOLOGY

There is no agreed Chinese translation of the term 'dyslexia'. The more common translations are: 'reading disability', 'literacy disability', and 'reading disorder'. Difference in research objectives and goals may result in different usage or definition for the children with such problems. In Taiwan the term dyslexia does not often appear in academic research work mostly because the scholars who research pertinent subjects are in the field of special education and examine the question of reading and writing from an educational point of view by using the term 'reading disabilities'. The definition of reading disabilities is mostly the same as dyslexia in the following aspects: (1) intelligence is average or above average; (2) poor performance in reading; and (3) excluding the unfavourable factor of senses, emotional disabilities, and culture.

These terminologies may be significant in academic research, but in the practice of education, dyslexia is not separated from the main category of learning disability. In this chapter, it is within the category of 'literacy disability' when discussing the research of dyslexia, whereas when discussing related educational service and support systems, it comes within the category of 'learning disability'.

RESEARCH

The statistical data show that before 1995 research in dyslexia in this country was quite sporadic (16 papers), most of theses written by graduate students. After 1995, the number of research papers suddenly increased greatly (91 papers). These include 26 master's theses and doctoral dissertations, and 30 papers from the special research project of the National Science Foundation. However, there are only four papers about writing disability. The more common research methods used are correlation and comparison research, but experimental research, case investigation research, longitudinal research, and cross-research are not sufficient (Chung-Chu Wang, 2001). Most of the researchers specialize in the field of

International Book of Dyslexia: A Guide to Practice and Resources. Edited by Ian Smythe, John Everatt and Robin Salter. ISBN 0-471-49646-4. © 2004 John Wiley & Sons, Ltd.

special education, with some in psychology, and few in the medical profession. This tendency seems quite different from other countries.

PREVALENCE OF DYSLEXIA

In 1978, Wei-Fan Kao was the first man to investigate the students in Taipei, Hualien, and Kaoshiung, and he found that only 2.91 per cent of students seemed to have dyslexia. But in 1982, Stevenson *et al.* carried out a cross-study of students in Taiwan, the USA, and Japan, and discovered 7.5 per cent of students in Taiwan had dyslexia, which was statistically close to the cross-study average of 6.3 per cent. It indicates the occurrence rate is not significantly affected by the difference in language writing systems.

LEGISLATION

In 1977, 'special education practice guidelines' began to include learning disability for special education service purposes, and thus learning disability was formally included in the special education service by law. After the Special Education Law was passed in 1984, dyslexia began to be protected by law like other disabilities, and students are entitled to have the right of receiving special education. In 1992, the government proclaimed, 'The criteria for examining students with language disability, physical weakness, abnormal personality, and multiple disabilities, and guidelines for educational assistance', thus, the definition of learning disability and its examination were formally presented (Li-yu Hung, 1995).

A learning disability is not listed under The Protection Law of Physical and Mental Disability, though the right to education of persons with learning disability is protected by the Special Education Law, but their survival rights are not protected by protection laws.

ADMINISTRATION

In Taiwan, the Ministry of Education takes charge of education, as well as the Bureau of Education in cities and counties. In the early years, special education was not separate from other educational affairs. In 1997, the Ministry of Education set up a Special Education Group to handle special education affairs. Starting in 1999, the Special Education Division for Special Educational Affairs was set up in cities and counties. The organization of a special education division has been instrumental in ensuring that the rights of students with learning disability are respected. With assistance coming from scholars, some cities and counties have been training special education and general education teachers in learning disability. Thanks to the programme, 'learning disability' is not a foreign term to school teachers now.

ASSESSMENT

Assessment of learning disability can be done by doctors in the departments of psychiatry and children's mental intelligence in hospitals. At school, assessment can be done by the Committee for Examining and Assisting Students in Need of Special Education.

Students are entitled to receive special education services after being assessed by the committee.

Members of the above committee include medical professionals, special education scholars, and learning disability parents' groups. At present, the criteria for the examination of learning disability are: intelligence test, learning achievement test, and the observation reports from teachers and parents. The lack of instruments in examination poses a problem for the concerned committee. From 1997 to 1999, the Ministry of Education compiled all related research work into 'instruments for examining students with learning disability', and there are 13 instruments for examining different cognitive abilities. These are the generally accepted instruments in examination.

RE-PLACEMENT CHOICES

In Taiwan the re-placement choices for students with learning disability are: a special education school, a special education class, or resource classes. A city or county government's budget and judgement of the value of special education may determine the number of resource classes. With limited resource classes in some cities and counties, most of the students with learning disability are still placed in general classes, not receiving any special education service. In Taipei and Kaoshung, the two big centrally-governed cities, every elementary school and junior high school has at least one resource class, offering a better service for students with a learning disability.

Most resource classes are not divided into different learning groups, and in them there are students with learning disability and other students with physical or mental disability. Teachers may teach them in separate groups.

Besides general public or private schools, there is no special school for learning disability or dyslexia in Taiwan. The parents have no other place to try teaching for learning disability outside the normal school system.

INSTRUCTION

At present in Taiwan there are no textbooks to improve reading and writing for students with dyslexia, nor are there technical assistance tools on the market. In addition to the market factor, scholars of the theory of 'sensory integration' have misled the general public and made the parents and teachers believe that the method of 'sensory integration' may 'cure' disability and thus have delayed the writing of textbooks.

At present the teaching of students with learning disability is mostly carried out in schools. In the past, a remediation teaching strategy to help students catch up with the normal students was carried out in the resource class, with no further teaching to increase the reading and writing ability of students with dyslexia. Teachers in general classes were not able to provide individual instruction for students with dyslexia. In recent years, after teachers have been professionally trained, some of them have created techniques and textbooks based on academic theories to improve the students' reading and writing ability.

ACCOMMODATION SERVICES

As specified in the Special Education Law, the school should provide students with learning disability with an assistance service, in which the following are offered to the students with reading and writing disability: a recording and reading service, a notetaking service, and computer assistance. Whether a teacher in a general or resource class has a good understanding of reading and writing disability may determine the services they provide for the students. Most students with dyslexia have not received adequate service.

For the admission tests to high schools and universities, there have been cases that provided reading service and extended test time for students with dyslexia. But at present the reading service is provided for a group, not on an individual basis. So far, there is no accommodation service for students with a learning disability while taking admission tests to universities. According to the legal guidelines for assisting students with physical and mental disability to complete compulsory education, the students with learning disability may have an extra 25 per cent added to their score. Protected by the policy, they are placed in general or vocational schools.

ADVOCACY GROUPS

In June 1996, the Parents' Association for Learning Disability in Taipei was founded, to ensure the education rights of the students with learning disability are respected. In December 1997, the Learning Disability Association in Taiwan was founded.

The founding of the private advocacy groups has united the power of parents and awakened the general public to a better understanding of children with a learning disability, and therefore helps them to respect their rights to education. Also through the published materials, the information has become easily available to more people.

Besides the Learning Disability Association in Taiwan as a national association, there are the Parents' Association for Learning Disability in Taipei, the Learning Disability Association in Ilan, and the Learning Disability Education Association in Hsin Chu. In addition to these, the Learning Disability Association in Kaoshung and the Learning Disability Association in Taoyuan are being set up. All these associations will work together for children with a learning disability.

ORGANIZATIONS

Learning Disability Association in Taiwan
Tel.: (04)23505899
Fax: (04)23505805
Email: ocd100229@ms36.hinet.net
Website: www.dale.nhctc.edu.tw/ald

Parents' Association for Learning Disability (in Taipei)
Tel.: (02)27099796
Fax: (02)27099801
Email: p7840109@ms27.hinet.net

Learning Disability Education Association in Hsin Chu
Tel.: (03)5722136

Learning Disability Association in Ilan
Tel.: (03)9575124

CHAPTER AUTHOR

Wei-Pai Blanche Lue
10F-3, No. 1–30
Syi-Ping So. Ln
Syi-Tun Road
Sec 3
Taichung
Taiwan
R. O. C.
Email: blanche-lue@hotmail.com

DYSLEXIA IN THAILAND

Jareeluk Jiraviboon

INTRODUCTION

Special education in Thailand was originally provided for the blind, deaf and mentally retarded through the encouragement of the King. Few people heard about learning disabilities at that time. Learning disabilities became well known in 1992 thanks to the National Education Act and later with the introduction of the special education section in the National Education Act (1999). Many departments of education are interested in special education, especially learning disabilities.

PROVISION OF SPECIAL EDUCATION IN THAILAND

Chapter 2, 'Educational Rights and Duties' in the National Education Act of Thailand of 1999 emphasized special education for people with physical, mental, intellectual, emotional, social, communication, and learning deficiencies, i.e. those with physical disabilities. This included those unable to support themselves, or those destitute or disadvantaged who should all have the rights and opportunities to receive the basic education specially provided. Education for the disabled shall be provided free of charge at birth or at first diagnosis. The Ministry of Education established the policy that in 2002 all children shall receive compulsory education for the duration of at least nine years. In 1999 the Ministry of Education implemented programmes according to the policy on education for people with special needs for educational opportunities to participate in the integrated programme in primary schools. So special education has become an important issue.

The Office of the National Primary Education Commission (ONPEC) is the important office of education in Thailand. ONPEC has decentralized the provision of special education to all 76 provinces. The offices of provincial primary education in co-operation with the offices of district primary education, 'school clusters' and schools are responsible for the development of special education. One school in each school cluster acts as an academic centre for special education as well as a venue for children with special needs

International Book of Dyslexia: A Guide to Practice and Resources. Edited by Ian Smythe, John Everatt and Robin Salter. ISBN 0-471-49646-4. © 2004 John Wiley & Sons, Ltd.

to attend the integration programme. ONPEC supports the provision of special education by the following methods:

- ONPEC allocates 300 baht or more to each student with special needs; leading schools, which provide special education, are allocated 53,200–130,000 baht to build academic support rooms (41 baht = 1 dollar US);
- to develop personnel, ONPEC provides training courses for special education teachers (200 hours);
- encouraging each school to make one school an academic centre for special education and a venue for children attending the integration programme;
- publishing documents on special education and disseminating them to all schools;
- purchasing 4,221 training kits (14 books per each training kit) for schools which are academic centres for special education;
- exhibiting special education: learning reform for the new millennium.

DYSLEXIA IN THAILAND

In order to provide a special education service, many teachers are interested in special education. They want to know more about it; about the characteristics of students with special needs and the way to diagnose and teach these children. It has been found that 14 per cent of students in primary school are students with learning disabilities and no less than 6 per cent are dyslexic.

Although few teachers had heard about 'dyslexia', for a long time in primary school, there were a lot of problems with the academic performance of students. The important problem was they were unable to read, some could not read aloud or tell the story after reading; some could not write complex words, some failed on reading comprehension. Teachers wanted to know the reasons for the failure in academic performance. Some teachers assumed failure was because of the low IQ of their students, because of low attention in learning to read, or because of inappropriate teaching methods. Most under-achieving students could not read and had low self-esteem. So teachers tried to help them to gain success in reading by remedial teaching. For example, if there was a student who was unable to read, teachers would collect the student's workbooks, test his or her reading skill, observe his or her learning style and discuss ideas for helping the student. Then the teacher would teach the student how to read by using the best way.

Most teachers in primary school use direct instruction to teach phonic skills for reading and spelling to students with reading disabilities. They taught students individually in their free time – maybe in the morning before class, after lunch or while waiting for parents in the afternoon. Some students got better at reading while some students were still unsuccessful. Many Thai people say that it is not easy to read the Thai language. It is a complex language with 44 letters, 32 vowels and 5 tonal accents. The Thai language has many synonymous words and homonymous words, and many idioms. So not many students succeed at reading.

A CASE STUDY OF DYSLEXIA

In 1995 I was the director of 'The Helping Slow Learners Project' in a primary school. The main object of this project was to help the students to learn in appropriate forms in accordance with their competencies and to give them a good attitude to learning. At that time, there was a dyslexic 9-year-old student in Grade 1 who had problems remembering the words he had just read. He could not read or write complex words. The first step to help him was setting an individual education plan (IEP) for him in collaboration with his teachers and his parents. I taught him through the multi-sensory approach. Art and music were always used in this practice too. He learned to read and write every morning, Monday to Friday. At first I taught phonic skills for reading and spelling, but he could not spell aloud. He surprised me by writing correct words in dictation. So I taught him by the whole words and multi-sensory approach. I let him see words in his favourite stories. He wrote and read many times through playing games with me or playing alone. It worked. He could match words and sound. He could read without spelling the words aloud. He could read and write complex words that he had selected. I felt good to know that he was happy in reading. His parents were satisfied with his success in reading although he could not spell aloud. He told me that he wanted to learn more and more. In my opinion, it is good to start learning to read with a good attitude and happy feelings.

It was my first case of dyslexia. He is my inspiration in teaching students with LD. Now I always teach by the multi-sensory approach and play method.

Finally, I think that if teaching dyslexia in the world is like a man, teaching dyslexia in Thailand seems to be a baby. He will grow up in his context. Teachers, parents, friends and society will help him to be a useful man in the future. I have told many teachers that it may be difficult in the beginning but when you see a little boy grow up to be a smart man, you will be happy.

CHAPTER AUTHOR

Jareeluk Jiraviboon
900/319 Udomsuk
26 Sukhumvit
103 Bangna
Bangkok 10260
Thailand
Email: jareeluk@yahoo.com

DYSLEXIA IN TOBAGO

Helen Sunderland

INTRODUCTION

Before April 2000 there was no provision for assessment or diagnosis of dyslexia in Tobago, for adults or children. Families who suspected their child might be dyslexic had to travel to Trinidad (overnight by boat or a short but expensive plane journey) and pay for a private diagnosis. However, even with a diagnosis, there was no provision in Tobago for specialist support for dyslexia or for the training of teachers in the area of dyslexia. In general, public awareness of the facts and issues surrounding dyslexia was low.

In April 2000 the Tobago Literacy Unit (TLU) was developed out of what had previously been ALTA Tobago and some of the issues began to be addressed. The TLU put on a ten-day training programme for 46 teachers and workers in the community (for instance, the children's librarian) which encompassed dyslexia awareness and support for children and adults with poor literacy skills. It also commissioned a consultancy on dyslexia. Both the training and consultancy were carried out by staff from the London Language and Literacy Unit (LLLU) at South Bank University, London, and were funded by BP Amoco.

Following the consultancy, the TLU decided to set up a Dyslexia Unit specifically to support dyslexic learners. The Unit would provide diagnosis and support for both children and adults. Staff from the Unit would also work in schools and would carry out dyslexia awareness training with school teachers, parents and other community workers. However, until funding for the Unit could be found, some support for dyslexic learners was set up at the TLU. This started immediately after the April 2000 training and is still ongoing.

Seed funding has just been granted by the J.B. Fernandes Trust to set up the Tobago Dyslexia Unit (TDU) and it is hoped that the work will then be carried forward by the Tobago Education Division with some funding coming through training in other islands. Talks are currently underway with the Education Division. The TLU has obtained

International Book of Dyslexia: A Guide to Practice and Resources. Edited by Ian Smythe, John Everatt and Robin Salter. ISBN 0-471-49646-4. © 2004 John Wiley & Sons, Ltd.

additional space for the TDU which comprises an assessment room, a classroom and a library. The Dyslexia Unit became operational in January 2002.

LEGISLATION AND POLICIES

There is presently no legislation nor policies specifically to do with dyslexia. However, talks are currently taking place between the TLU and the Education Division.

IDENTIFICATION AND ASSESSMENT

As yet, there is no facility for identification and assessment in Tobago. However, this is one of the functions of the TDU. There is still a great deal of work to be done to establish local norms.

At present most tutors are not trained to give a full assessment. However, they have been trained in the use of some tools to give initial assessment for support purposes. These are as follows:

- a dyslexia screening test;
- an in-depth diagnostic interview;
- phonological and memory tests;
- single word and non-word reading tests;
- a spelling error analysis.

A core group of dyslexia tutors who have all attended initial training has been formed. They can carry out the above initial assessments to give an initial diagnosis, mainly for support purposes. They will make up the core staff at the Dyslexia Unit and will meet regularly to discuss issues arising from support and assessment. They will be supported by some tutor/managers who are fully trained in dyslexia assessment and support.

INTERVENTION AND RESOURCES

Some support for dyslexic learners, both adults and children, has been carried out at the TLU. Now that the Dyslexia Unit is formed, support is provided on the Dyslexia Unit's premises. Students with indicators of dyslexia will initially be given one-to-one support. This will last for at least 6–10 weeks to enable them to gain confidence and make some progress and to enable them to begin to understand their strengths and weaknesses and their own learning style. Once they have gained this initial understanding and confidence, they will be encouraged to join a group.

Initially all support will be provided on the premises of the Dyslexia Unit in order that tutors can build up experience and expertise. Assessment tools, teaching materials and reference books will all be kept there.

Once tutors have begun to feel confident in working with dyslexic students, the Dyslexia Unit will develop work with schools. It intends to start by setting up projects in one primary school and one secondary school to help support dyslexic students and their parents.

Teaching methods are targeted at students' strengths and weaknesses, and individual learning styles. They include:

- discussion of and understanding of the student's individual learning style;
- a metacognitive approach so that students understand how good learners learn and why they are having difficulty with certain tasks;
- a multi-sensory approach;
- overlearning and practice;
- a spelling programme using the 'look, say, cover, write, check' approach;
- a reading programme emphasizing high interest materials and good comprehension;
- use of models and writing frames for free writing;
- study and organization skills, e.g. colour coding, mind-mapping, personal mnemonics;
- preparation for autonomous/independent learning.

Funding has been granted by BP Amoco for the development and publication of reading booklets with a Caribbean focus for use in family learning and dyslexia support classes.

TEACHER TRAINING

In April 2000, staff from the London Language and Literacy Unit (LLLU) at London's South Bank University (SBU) ran a ten-day training programme for teachers and community workers which included dyslexia awareness, some initial assessment techniques and teaching strategies to support learners with poor literacy skills. Following this programme one TLU tutor took the Dyslexia Institute course in Trinidad and others started to run dyslexia support classes through the TLU.

In July 2001, the staff from the LLLU at SBU returned and ran more training – revision for those who attended the first course and training for new tutors. They also ran 'training the trainers' courses for TLU staff who wished to run dyslexia awareness training in the community.

These community courses are planned to start soon and will be targeted at parents, community workers and school teachers. The TLU will accredit its staff through the UK Open College Network and is currently working with the LLLU at SBU to develop the accreditation.

In the future, the TLU hopes to be able to offer training in adult literacy and dyslexia awareness and support to interested persons and organizations throughout the eastern Caribbean. This is one way of becoming self-supporting in the long term.

ADVOCACY GROUPS

The TLU currently acts as an advocacy group for dyslexic learners. It has organized meetings between parents and TLU staff, and the consultants from LLLU at SBU. It has also done much to raise awareness about dyslexia on the island, for instance, appearing on Tobago radio and talking at organizations such as the Tobago Rotary Club. The Tobago Information Unit has expressed interest in filming sessions with TLU which will include understanding and supporting persons with dyslexia. This will raise awareness in the community and publicize good practice in working with dyslexic learners.

It also plans to run dyslexia awareness sessions for schools and communities in locations throughout the island.

EXAM AND CURRICULUM PROVISIONS

The new Dyslexia Unit will be responsible for negotiating special considerations for dyslexic candidates with examination boards.

ADULT PROVISIONS

Adult learners of literacy are supported through the Tobago Literacy Unit classes. These take place at the TLU's headquarters in Scarborough, the capital, and also in community locations throughout the island. All TLU tutors are currently trained in dyslexia awareness and support, and the TLU will be adding units on dyslexia to its Tutor Training Programme so that new tutors will also receive training. Dyslexic adults will be able to receive assessment and support on an individual basis through the new Dyslexia Unit so that they are able to make progress and develop an understanding of their learning style before they progress on to a TLU course.

CHAPTER AUTHOR

Helen Sunderland
35 Fernside Rd
London SW12 8LN
Email: Helenlllu@cocoon.co.uk

Dyslexia in the USA

Jane Browning

INTRODUCTION

To attempt to explain how dyslexia is currently addressed in the United States is, to say the least, daunting. There are national and state laws involved, that both provide services, and also offer protection against discrimination. There has been extensive research into reading and dyslexia in the past 20 years that has greatly influenced views of reading disabilities in the United States. In addition, the issue of appropriate means of teaching children to read has become a major agenda item of President Bush. He made the issue of 'reading' a major campaign item ('reading is the new civil right') and has made the idea of 'No child left behind' the cornerstone of his education reform efforts.

Few professionals in the field of reading in the United States have a grasp of all the key elements identified from the research. Despite the efforts of advocacy groups, and funded 'protection and advocacy organizations', the average parent or the adult with dyslexia is often placed in a position of trying to find services without very much understanding of the problem, or the laws. There is even less understanding of the access to research on literacy issues. Although the Internet has greatly improved access to information, schools fail to respond to laws and research.

The situation is complicated by the fact that each state can have a different standard on dyslexia and therefore a different standard for who does and does not get help. (A joke in the United States is that the best way to fix a learning disability is to cross a state line.) However, some of this problem is addressed in the new 'No Child Left Behind' Education Bill of 2001, in which states are now to be held accountable for the reading success of all students.

LEARNING DISABILITIES

In the United States, the term learning disabilities (LD) is not the same as used in England and many other countries. The term was developed in the early 1960s to differentiate

International Book of Dyslexia: A Guide to Practice and Resources. Edited by Ian Smythe, John Everatt and Robin Salter. ISBN 0-471-49646-4. © 2004 John Wiley & Sons, Ltd.

between those who were of 'average and above average' intelligence and those of 'low' intelligence, having severe reading problems.

In the ensuing years, the term LD has come to include persons, with a presumed central nervous system disorder, having difficulty in reading, writing and mathematics. While there are many definitions of LD, almost all include dyslexia as a subset, but to complicate matters, many parents do not consider dyslexia as a learning disability.

PREVALENCE

Currently about 10 per cent of the school age population in the United States are considered to have disabilities, and qualify for Special Education Services; one-half of these students are classified as having LD. The latest studies funded by the National Institute of Health (1995) show that about 85 per cent of those with LD have reading disabilities, or what is considered in a broad sense, dyslexia. If recognized with disabilities, children are covered against discrimination by the federal law (The Rehabilitation Act of 1973, specifically, Section 504). However, special educational services for these children are required and provided through another federal law, the Individuals with Disabilities Education Act (IDEA). This law was mainly designed to address the long-term avoidance of public schools in providing education for children with physical disabilities in the least restricted environment, the classroom. The advocates for persons with LD wanted to focus on the needs of children with dyslexia to have reading training in 'resource rooms' or in breakout sessions. This conflict over the 'least restrictive environment' and 'inclusion' continues to cause disunity in the special education community.

While identified children with dyslexia face the problem of inappropriate services from ill-trained teachers, many more face the problem of no services at all. While 5 per cent of children are classified as having LD, NICHD research has shown that up to 17 per cent of children have a reading disorder that could be called dyslexia. This means that as many as two-thirds of dyslexics are not identified in schools. This is a major concern that the 'No child left behind' legislation and approach are attempting to address.

In the past several years, as special education costs have skyrocketed, there has been a greater push towards 'full inclusion' and more requirements have been put upon the classroom teacher to provide reading instructions for children with dyslexia. At the same time, teachers were told to use 'whole language' approaches to teaching. While in the late 1970s many school districts attempted to use multi-sensory phonic-based programmes developed by the Slingerland Institute and the Orton Dyslexia Society, by the 1990s most of these efforts had been abandoned.

Most experts in LD saw whole language as one of the least appropriate ways of teaching dyslexics. The US Department of Education, first under the Clinton administration, and now wholeheartedly under the Bush administration, has moved towards the views of most experts in the area of dyslexia. Through extensive publications and now, legislation, the US government is supporting the incorporation of the approaches towards reading pioneered in the dyslexic community and supported by the research of the National Institute of Health's National Institute of Child and Human Development (NICHD). The findings of what was named the 'National Reading Panel,' are being recommended by the Bush administration, not just for children with learning disabilities, but for all children, and starting at a very early age (pre-school and kindergarten). New funds are being authorized for extensive teacher training in these approaches. In addition, for the first time in the nation's history, all schools will need to have a standardized reading test for ALL students, not as a means of measuring a student's failure, but as a means to identify schools that are failing to provide appropriate teaching.

THE IDEA LAW

The overall hope is that through very early intervention, with research-based methods, the number of those who have reading failure, due to dyslexia or other reasons, will be greatly reduced, as would be the number of those in need of services under special education pro-grammes. Under IDEA, the services are costly (three to four times the cost for non-disabled children). The states bear about 85 per cent of the costs of services, while the federal government provides 15 per cent.

To qualify for IDEA services, a student must be identified as having a learning disability through the use of an inter-disciplinary team, and professional evaluators The team, plus parents, then develops an individual education programme (IEP). This plan includes all the interventions and remediation approaches that will be provided for the child. Some schools also include a '504' plan to deal with accommodation approaches in the general classroom (such as taking tests in isolation, having oral exams, or being provided with books on tape) as a separate process, apart from the IEP approach.

The process in schools of gaining identification for IDEA is very complex and time-consuming. Often the diagnosis is poorly done by schools and parents who have the resources challenge the diagnosis, adding to the overall costs of 'special education'. These challenges often have to be done over and over again as the child changes teachers or schools. This has led to many parents seeking added support outside of schools or giving up entirely on public schools.

PRIVATE TUITION

Parents often have to seek diagnostic testing outside school. This can cost from US$600 to US$2,000. They also seek tutors trained in such programmes as the Slingerland/Orton or Orton/Gillingham methods of teaching reading. The fees tends to be in the US$30–60 per hour range, but vary by location and demand. In most cases, public schools traditionally do not pay for this type of service.

For those who give up on the public schools, there is in most major cities in the United States at least one, often many, private school designed specifically for children with LD or dyslexia. These types of schools are rarer in smaller cities and rural areas. While these schools tend to be expensive (US$10–25,000 a year in tuition), many have working arrangements by which public schools, who are obligated to provide services under IDEA, pay the tuition.

One more layer of service is available through a small number of private boarding or preparatory schools that are generally small and very costly. They tend to serve mainly boys. Most of these schools are concentrated in the New York/New England area, and are not as accessible to parents throughout the rest of the nation.

While this chapter has made an attempt to show the state of dyslexia in the United States, it has not addressed the issues of adults, nor discussed the major national organizations addressing the issue, such as the Learning Disabilities Association of America, the International Dyslexia Association, the National Center on Learning Disabilities, the Schwab Foundation, and many others.

CONCLUSION

The situation for LD and dyslexics is complex, which has contributed to the high incidence of failure – only 30 per cent of those with LD receive a standard high school diploma. The need is very clear for raising standards by the new 'No child left behind' education reform now being introduced.

ORGANIZATIONS

Learning Disabilities Association of America
4156 Library Road
Pittsburgh
PA 15234-1349
USA
Tel.: (412) 341-1515
Email: info@ldaamerica.org
Website: www.ldaamerica.org

International Dyslexia Association
Chester Building Suite 382
8600 La Salle Road
Baltimore
MD 21286 2044
Maryland
USA
Website: www.interdys.org

CHAPTER AUTHOR

Jane Browning
Executive Director of the Learning Disabilities Association of America
4156 Library Road
Pittsburgh
PA 15234-1349
USA
Email: jbrowning@ldaamerica.org

DYSLEXIA IN WALES

Ann Cooke

INTRODUCTION

Wales, a country in the western part of the United Kingdom, has distinctive cultural and linguistic characteristics and geographical features that give it a unique identity. The region is small, about 120 miles from north to south, and about 90 miles from east to west at its widest part, with a population of 4.5 million. It is a land of mountains and uplands, highest in the north and mid-Wales, with the largest centres of population in the valleys and coastal plain of the south. The cultural heritage of Wales is to be found in its Welsh language, which is quite different from English (though the alphabets are similar). Welsh and English have equal status as official languages of Wales. Just under 20 per cent of people in Wales speak Welsh as their first language, and are fully bilingual, with a command of literacy in both languages. The proportion of Welsh speakers varies regionally; the highest proportion of those speaking Welsh as their first language live in the northern and western areas.

Constitutionally, Wales is part of the UK but it has had, since 1997, a partially devolved government. People in Wales elect members Members of Parliament in the UK system; they also elect members of the Welsh Assembly, which has its seat in the capital city, Cardiff, in the south of the country. The Welsh Assembly is responsible for implementing government policy and statutes originating in the UK Parliament. Though it is not a fully legislative body, it creates Welsh policy within the devolved system, and adapts certain aspects of legislation to the particular needs and characteristics of Wales.

Education is a major responsiblity of the Welsh Assembly. Education legislation comes into force after revision to meet the circumstances and needs of children and schools in Wales. Accordingly, the National Curriculum, which prescribes the content and structure of what is taught, and the Code of Practice, which sets out the way that legislation on the education of children with special needs should be implemented, both have their equivalent Welsh versions. Due to the rural nature of Wales, some primary schools have fewer

International Book of Dyslexia: A Guide to Practice and Resources. Edited by Ian Smythe, John Everatt and Robin Salter. ISBN 0-471-49646-4. © 2004 John Wiley & Sons, Ltd.

than 30 children. The educational needs of dyslexic children in Wales must be seen within this framework.

THE EDUCATIONAL SYSTEM

Education in Wales conforms broadly to the same Education Acts and policy as that of England. The ages for compulsory education are the same (5 to 16), the curriculum follows the same stages as in England, and the assessment and examination systems are similar. The policy of inclusion in which (with the exception of certain groups with severe difficulties or particular disabilities), all children attend the same, mainstream school, is part of the ethos of education. This implies that every teacher has responsibility for teaching children with all kinds of special need, dyslexia included. Among schools the systems vary: in some (especially in secondary schools), children with special needs in literacy, and possibly numeracy, may be taught in special groups; in some counties, between 1 per cent and 3 per cent of children across the age-range may be withdrawn for individual tuition.

The framework for setting out provision for the needs of individuals is to be found in the Welsh Code of Practice, 2002. This identifies three distinct ways in which needs may be met: (1) support within the school; (2) within the school but with a contribution from external agencies; and (3) enhanced provision under a Statement of Special Need for children with complex or very severe difficulties.

Children with difficulties are usually noticed first by the class teacher, though parents often ask for a particular check to be made. An informal assessment will be made by the school's co-ordinator for special needs and thereafter by an advisory teacher. Following this kind of identification, an Individual Education Plan will be drawn up and put into practice. If the child's progress is not satisfactory after a stated time, he or she may be referred for further, more searching assessment by an educational psychologist.

THE WELSH LANGUAGE IN EDUCATION

Welsh is a core (essential) subject of the National Curriculum for all children in Wales. It may be taught as a first, or as a second language. For Welsh-speaking children in Welsh-medium schools, English is introduced formally into the curriculum after school year 2. Throughout Wales, Welsh is introduced as an oral language for English-speaking children from the early years. In some counties, especially in North and West Wales, it is also the medium of instruction for all children in the early years and this includes the introduction to reading and writing. The general objective is that children should be bilingual orally, and on the way to command of the second language in its written form, by the time they are 11. They have therefore two languages to master.

IDENTIFYING DYSLEXIA IN WALES AND IN CHILDREN LEARNING IN WELSH

Welsh has a very regular phonic spelling system so that it is possible for most children to make a start with reading and writing as soon as they know the alphabet. It has sometimes been assumed that children taught in Welsh would be less likely to experience dyslexia-type difficulties, and this may be partly true. However, it has tended to hinder the early identification of dyslexia, especially among children whose first language is Welsh. When given a reading and spelling test in Welsh, these children may perform within the average band. Their difficulties do not become apparent until reading and writing are introduced in English. It has sometimes been assumed, therefore, that the difficulties are produced by the linguistic situation and that, with time, they will disappear.

There is no reason to suppose that the incidence of dyslexia is lower in Wales than elsewhere. Early screening materials for dyslexia are available (in English only at present) but identification of dyslexia is more likely to be based on attainment in reading and spelling than on the use of special diagnostic tests. For children learning in Welsh, reading and spelling tests need to be sensitive to the way that dyslexia difficulties affect the learning of literacy in Welsh. For instance, the written grammar of Welsh may be more likely to produce errors than the spelling. After identification, teaching materials and reading books for Welsh dyslexic children also need to be sensitive to the characteristics of the language, and to the way that dyslexia may affect bilingual learning.

TRAINING OF TEACHERS

If children with dyslexia are to learn in an inclusive education system in Wales, all teachers must be aware of the way that dyslexia presents in the two languages, and of appropriate ways to help them. Initial teacher training courses provide a brief introduction to dyslexia and information about how children may be helped in class. For qualified teachers, short in-service courses, and more specialized professional development courses are all available in Wales. However, local education policies on dyslexia, and training opportunities, differ from one county to another. In general, it is accepted that all schools should have at least one teacher who has taken, if not a fully accredited training course in dyslexia, at least an enhanced awareness course.

LEARNING SUPPORT ASSISTANTS

In many schools Learning Support Assistants (LSAs) are employed to give individual support to children in the classroom, and this may be critical for successful inclusion of children with learning difficulties and disabilities. While LSAs are not trained teachers, opportunities for professional training for this role are increasing, in Wales as elsewhere. Here again, it is essential that there should be understanding of how dyslexia affects children's learning in Welsh schools, and in the bilingual situation.

COURSES FOR TEACHERS

Part-time Master's and Certificate courses for teachers wishing to specialize in dyslexia work are offered at institutions in both North and South Wales. These draw students from all over the UK and also internationally; two have attracted students especially from Ireland and Greece. Local Education Authorities (LEAs) have also taken the initiative for setting up courses, and for the development of courses for Learning Support Assistants.

All these courses conform to British Dyslexia Association (BDA) criteria for specialist dyslexia courses, and teachers completing them are eligible to apply for BDA Accredited

Teacher Status (40-hour courses) or Associate Membership (AMBDA) (90-hour courses including a unit or module on assessment).

EARLY WORK ON DYSLEXIA IN WALES

Pioneer work has gone on in Wales both in research into dyslexia and in provision of help for children assessed as dyslexic. The work of Professor Tim Miles on assessment, which led to his Bangor Dyslexia Test, was carried out in the Department of Psychology, University of Wales, Bangor, in the 1960s and 1970s. Following on from this work, help from specially trained teachers was offered to local schools. In 1974 this help was adopted by the Education Authority in the county of Gwynedd as their provision for dyslexic children with the most severe difficulties. From the outset, there has been awareness that children whose first language is Welsh may need an approach tailored to their particular linguistic needs. A programme of teaching, based on her own work and that of colleagues, was produced by a Bangor teacher (*O Gam i Gam – From Step to Step*).

Particular emphasis at Bangor has been on the development of understanding about the needs of dyslexic individuals in further and higher education, and ways to address their difficulties. Help for dyslexic students in the university began to be given in Bangor in the 1970s and the Bangor support service has been used as a model by a number of institutions of higher education in the UK.

DIVERSITY OF PROVISION FOR SCHOOL-AGE PUPILS

While the Gwynedd/Bangor approach to intervention favoured a general policy of withdrawal for one-to-one teaching, continuing for several years, in other centres different policies have been adopted. In a secondary school in Hawarden, Flintshire, a whole-school policy was developed which depended on class and subject teachers being aware of the needs of dyslexic pupils, and helping them within their subject specialisms. Specialist help for the development of literacy and numeracy skills was available within the school.

Such whole-school policies for children in the 11–16 age group were adopted elsewhere, while teaching in small groups was more often to be found in use for children in primary schools. The establishment of centres for specialist teaching was a third option, usually to be found where clusters of primary schools made attendance for part of the day possible without the need for extra lengthy travelling. Particular LEAs have responded to needs according to regional geography and the size of schools.

The contribution of schools in the independent sector must not be ignored and two in particular have offered support for pupils with special needs and with dyslexia. The boarding situation of the schools enables provision to be made for particular interests, and for extra-curricular activities, that have made a significant contribution to success for many youngsters.

THE WELSH DYSLEXIA PROJECT

This not-for-profit organization was set up in 2001 to promote work on several aspects of dyslexia in Wales. As well as marking the beginning of important new developments, the

Welsh Dyslexia Project should help to consolidate and build on the provision and organizations that are already in place. Further details are given in the next chapter.

DYSLEXIA-FRIENDLY SCHOOL INITIATIVES

The dyslexia-friendly school project was launched by the BDA in 1996 and has been adopted by a number of LEAs, including some in Wales. Several counties have taken on board the ideas of this project, notably Swansea, where the policy is promoted in all schools by the Education Authority. In other areas, for instance, Flintshire, a 'bottom-up' model has been favoured, in which schools match their policy, practice and provision to a set of criteria and apply for the dyslexia-friendly school status. After that, the school is expected to show, through a system of internal and external monitoring, that it continues to put the agreed standards into practice.

While the expectations are similar in both models, one is county-driven, the other is an 'opt-in' approach. In both approaches, the effects should be that pupils with dyslexia are identified early, and that their needs are understood and met throughout the curriculum. With a dyslexia-friendly policy in place, the numbers of children needing individual provision should be limited to those with the most severe difficulties. Above all, such a policy should mean that dyslexic pupils should experience school as a positive environment for learning, and thereby have better opportunities for success.

THE BDA IN WALES

Several local associations of the British Dyslexia Association are active in Wales, with one group covering north-west and north Wales, and several in the south. The smaller and more scattered populations of north and central Wales make frequent meetings difficult and day events, such as family days, bring in larger numbers. Many successful day conferences focusing on general issues and new developments have been run, for example, by the Dyslexia Unit (University of Wales, Bangor), in the north, and by the BDA and local associations in south and central Wales. In the south a rolling programme of meetings is more possible.

Geography and the absence of motorways linking north, central and south Wales mean that it has not, so far, been found practicable to set up a Welsh Dyslexia Association. Despite this, the Dyslexia Associations in Wales have well-established links with the BDA and individual parents can find advice and support from local befrienders. Many individuals have worked hard to improve awareness and provision for dyslexic children in Wales, and to provide a network for dyslexic adults.

ORGANIZATIONS

Prosiect Dyslexia Cymru/Welsh Dyslexia Project
For support in Welsh and English
Website: www.welshdyslexia.info
Email: llechryd@btinternet.com
Phone: 01239 682 849

Bangor Dyslexia Unit. University of Wales. Bangor
Website: http://www.dyslexia.bangor.ac.uk
Email: dyslex-admin@bangor.ac.uk
Phone: 01248 382 203

British Dyslexia Association. 98 London Road. Reading. RG1 5AU.
Website: www.bda-dyslexia.org.uk
Email: admin@bda-dyslexia.demon.co.uk
Phone: 0118 966 8271

CHAPTER AUTHOR

Ann Cooke
Dyslexia Unit
University of Wales
Bangor
Email: e.a.cooke@bangor.ac.uk

WELSH DYSLEXIA PROJECT/ PROSIECT DYSLECSIA CYMRU

Michael Davies and Ian Smythe

INTRODUCTION

The Welsh Dyslexia Project/Prosiect Dyslecsia Cymru (WDP/PDC) aims to bring together professionals working with the dyslexia community in Wales, the commercial sector, government agencies, parents and carers, as well as dyslexic individuals to create an environment where the dyslexic individual may develop their full potential. This will be facilitated through the development of awareness and understanding, as well as resources, for the support of the dyslexic individual.

The WDP recognizes the need to develop three principal areas:

- policies
- resources
- training.

The policies, through the Welsh Code of Practice, provide well-established principles. The WDP/PDC sees its role as ensuring the development of resources and training. If these are not being provided by government, service providers or others, the WDP/PDC will attempt to facilitate their development.

The aims and objectives which form the foundation of resource and service development of the WDP/PDC as set out in their strategic plan are presented below.

POLICIES

- Education policies should recognize that every individual has unique characteristics, interests, abilities and learning needs, and education systems should be designed to

International Book of Dyslexia: A Guide to Practice and Resources. Edited by Ian Smythe, John Everatt and Robin Salter. ISBN 0-471-49646-4. © 2004 John Wiley & Sons, Ltd.

provide informed evaluations and derive appropriate educational programmes to accommodate the wide diversity of these characteristics and needs.

- Work and life-related policies, e.g. disability discrimination legislation, should ensure that no individual is excluded or penalized because they learn in a different way.
- All policies should reflect that these rights are irrespective of the individual's first language.

RESOURCES

- A well researched, widely accepted test (or range of tests) for the screening and assessment of the dyslexic individual should be freely available for schools and EPs. These tests should provide the basis for the formation of an individual education plan, and/or guidance for personal development.
- Teaching and learning resources, e.g. paper and computer-based teaching materials, manuals, should be available to teach the dyslexic individual literacy and life skills.
- Support material and devices (e.g. text readers) should be widely accessible and acceptable for education and employment purposes.
- A central web-based resource centre is available to freely access additional material and information, as well as being a forum for further advice and sharing ideas.

EDUCATIONAL ESTABLISHMENTS AND EMPLOYERS

- Each educational establishment should have individuals (e.g. special educational needs co-ordinators) trained in the recognition of the dyslexic individual and their needs.
- All employers should be aware of the special needs and abilities of the dyslexic individual, and should ensure these abilities, strengths and weaknesses are fully utilized for the benefit of the individual, the employer and society.
- All staff should be trained in awareness and understanding of dyslexia, and how to accommodate the individual within the normal learning and working environment.
- All schools and employers should have policy guidelines to ensure an inclusive approach is adopted for dyslexia.
- Grievances procedures should be available, developed by the educational authorities/employer, which may arbitrate on any disputes.
- Any support provided should be seen as a fundamental human right, which ensures these individuals are empowered within society, and not perceived as an advantage.

TRAINING

- Every educational establishment should have staff trained in the identification of individuals with specific learning difficulties.
- All staff in educational establishments should be trained in the awareness and understanding of dyslexia, and how to accommodate this within a normal teaching environment.
- All others concerned with education (e.g. governors, learning support assistants and policy-makers) should know their responsibilities towards dyslexic individuals.

- All professionals working with dyslexic individuals (e.g. educational and occupational psychologists, speech and language therapists, disability officers) should be trained to identify specific learning difficulties.
- All those professionals dealing with human resources (e.g. personnel management) should be trained in the management and development of the dyslexic individual, as well as ensuring their rights are upheld.
- Every dyslexic individual should be provided with training to understand, discover, explore and capitalize upon their strengths and weaknesses.
- All parents of dyslexic children should be provided with training to understand the part they can play in the education of their child.

This statement of strategy has already led to the development of a series of resources and services, making Wales one of the most dyslexia-friendly countries in the world.

PROJECTS

The following projects have been completed (as at December 2002):

- a teacher-based screening tool for primary schools;
- dyslexia-friendly schools training;
- computer assessment for dyslexic adults, with webcam support;
- evaluation of software for adults in higher education;
- Web-based training for teachers, classroom assistants and parents;
- a Welsh website;
- teaching resources;
- a bilingual CD for parents of dyslexic children;
- a bilingual booklet for parents.

The WDP/PDC recognizes its support and inspiration from around the world, and in line with the philosophy of the late Marion Welchman, to whom the first *International Book of Dyslexia* was dedicated, we would be very happy to share our experience with all who ask. Further information may be found at www.welshdyslexia.info.

ORGANIZATION

Welsh Dyslexia Project/Prosiect Dyslecsia Cymru
Email: llechryd@btinternet.com
Website: www.welshdyslexia.info

CHAPTER AUTHORS

Michael Davies and Ian Smythe
Welsh Dyslexia Project
Llysteifi
Llechryd
Cardigan SA43 2NX
Email: ian.smythe@ukonline.co.uk

INDEX